**Handb**
**for De**

*An Evid*

MW00412437

# Handbook of Cognitive Hypnotherapy for Depression

## An Evidence-Based Approach

**Assen Alladin**
*Department of Psychology*
*Foothills Medical Centre*
*Calgary, Alberta*
*Canada*

Wolters Kluwer | Lippincott Williams & Wilkins
Health

Philadelphia · Baltimore · New York · London
Buenos Aires · Hong Kong · Sydney · Tokyo

*Acquisitions Editor:* Charley Mitchell
*Developmental Editor:* Jenny Koleth
*Project Manager:* Rosanne Hallowell
*Senior Manufacturing Manager:* Benjamin Rivers
*Marketing Manager:* Adam Glazer
*Design Coordinator and Cover Designer:* Terry Mallon
*Production Services:* Aptara, Inc.
*Printer:* R.R. Donnelley

**Library of Congress Cataloging-in-Publication Data**
Alladin, Assen.
  Handbook of cognitive hypnotherapy for depression : an evidence-based
approach / Assen Alladin.
    p. ; cm.
  Includes bibliographical references.
  ISBN-13: 978-0-7817-6604-3 (case)
  ISBN-10: 0-7817-6604-4 (case)
  1. Hypnotism—Therapeutic use—Handbooks, manuals, etc.  2. Depression,
Mental—Treatment—Handbooks, manuals, etc.  3. Cognitive theraphy—
Handbooks, manuals, etc.  4. Behavior therapy–Handbooks, manuals, etc. I. Title.
  [DNLM:  1. Dpressive Disorder—theraphy.  2. Cognitive Therapy—methods.
  3. Hypnosis. WM 171 A416h 2007]
  RC537.A4546 2007
  616.89′162—dc22

                                                          2006102068

                                        10  9  8  7  6  5  4  3  2  1

# Contents

# Foreword

I like to think of myself as an experienced and reasonably skillful clinician who frequently works successfully with depressed patients. I have even been accused of pulling rabbits out of hats to achieve certain positive clinical outcomes. Yet I have recently undergone a considerable growth experience. Its precipitant and medium was my reading Assen Alladin's *Handbook of Cognitive Hypnotherapy for Depression: An Evidence-Based Approach* from cover to cover. I will never again be able to look at depression the same way I viewed it before reading Dr. Alladin's remarkable book. In truth this book has already begun to exert its influence on my clinical practice, and I suspect the growth in me that it has promoted is far from finished.

Every major branch of the healing arts deals with the problem of depression, and, unfortunately, numerous modalities tend, at times, to compete with one another, each claiming to have the "right approach." Yet we know that depression is a multifaceted clinical illness that can have its roots in genetics, neurophysiology, family psychopathology, behavior patterns, false conceptions of the self and the world, trauma, and myriad other contributing causalities. It is indeed, as Dr. Alladin tells us, ". . . a complex heterogeneous disorder requiring multiple interventions."

*Handbook of Cognitive Hypnotherapy for Depression* is a comprehensive manual for the hypnotically facilitated psychotherapy of patients with depressive disorders. It can be utilized both by the experienced clinician as well as by those who are "just beginners." The scope of the book is impressive, and its material is presented in a building process that leads the reader through the most basic concepts into the most vital, practical, and innovative techniques for working with depression. Dr. Alladin presents the reader with a clear, up-to-date review of the nature and types of depression, theories about its etiology, and contemporary treatment modalities. He follows this with reviews of cognitive behavior therapy, of therapeutic applications of clinical hypnosis and of the efficacy of cognitive hypnotherapy for depression. In Chapter 4, he proposes his circular feedback model of depression (an extension of Beck's model) and discusses his own cognitive dissociative theory of depression. This latter model, still in process, is groundbreaking. It provides ways of understanding how certain hypnotic interventions can be therapeutic, and it also integrates cognitive behavioral concepts with those that come from a more psychodynamic/trauma/dissociation base. The "basic" material presented is rich, embedded in contemporary neurobiological studies, epidemiology, behavioral research, and the interplay of theories with clinical evidence.

Before he offers clinical techniques, Dr. Alladin makes it clear why case formulation is a necessary ingredient in treating depression. The clinical techniques that follow are creative, pioneering, and extremely valuable. They are given in the form of detailed instruction, scripts, and thorough reports of clinical material. First Aid for Depression, for example, is something every clinician needs to know. Dr. Aladdin follows his section on cognitive hypnotherapy with specific techniques for creating and strengthening antidepressive pathways. It is not enough for depressive symptoms to abate, says Dr. Alladin: New ways of thinking and coping and their attendant new neurophysiology must be developed to replace old depressive pathways. He gives clinicians techniques that patients can be taught to use for breaking ruminative patterns, for behavioral activation, and for the development of social skills and relapse prevention. Additionally, he shows how the usefulness of mindfulness techniques and the development of spiritual resources can play vital roles in the treatment of depressive disorders. He even evaluates the role of antidepressant medications and places them where they belong in the treatment of depression—among a number of adjunctive therapies that can contribute significantly to recovery.

This is a book that contains tremendous balance and the integration of many fields of endeavor. It balances theory with clinical approach, explanation with detailed clinical scripts, research with application, evidence with effectiveness, the general within the context of the individual. It integrates academic and research-based material with their practical implications with living, breathing human beings.

There are certain classics in the fields of psychotherapy and of hypnosis that are also landmarks of major paradigm shifts. Time will reveal Assen Alladin's *Handbook of Cognitive Hypnotherapy for Depression: An Evidence-Based Approach* to be such a book. What is truly remarkable about this work is that, while it is a bold, ground-breaking, and practical practice-based manual for dealing with patients who suffer from depression, all of the techniques are soundly grounded in research and well-reasoned theory. Dr. Alladin has moved hypnotically facilitated cognitive behavior therapy into the 21st century by adopting the framework of evidence-based practice, a synthesis of research-based efficacy studies and (also well-researched) effectiveness factors such as empathy, the therapeutic alliance, rapid symptom relief, and hope.

For clinical hypnosis books, this is a new territory that brings both head and heart, science and the art of therapy into the psychotherapy of the depressed patient. "Evidence-based" treatment (based on efficacy studies) represents the will of the health sciences to place themselves on a truly scientific basis. Nevertheless, the dominance of clinical work by the findings of such studies has attracted a great deal of criticism for a number of reasons. Efficacy studies can be flawed because of design problems and population selection issues as well as problems that are inherent in introducing measurements into complex systems. They also can be confounded by the presence of such factors as comorbidities, issues of relative degrees of refractoriness, and unacknowledged transtheoretical effectiveness factors. Unfortunately, increasing numbers of clinicians have been feeling that they might have to choose between manualized therapies and good, individualized clinical practice. Dr. Alladin's approach offers the new state of the art: psychotherapy that integrates science and the caring, attentive, and cooperating presence of the therapist into clinical practice. Although this book helps clinicians know a lot more about depression, it also emphasizes psychoeducation of the patient and the patient's self-care. It features "homework" in the forms of reporting, self-assessment, behavioral and self-hypnosis exercises, new activities, and so forth as part of the developing therapeutic alliance between patient and therapist, an alliance whose aim is to increase the patient's healthy autonomy.

I am grateful for the opportunity to participate in the launching of this unique and wonderful book. I have no doubt that the growth experience it has created within me (which is far from over) will be only one of a multitude that will take place among its readers.

*Claire Frederick, M.D.*
Tufts University School of Medicine
Boston, Massachusetts

*Dr. Claire Frederick is a psychiatrist who practices in Bangor, Maine, and Cambridge, Massachusetts. She is on the faculty of the Tufts University School of Medicine in Boston, and is Distinguished Consulting Faculty at the Saybrook School of Graduate Studies and Research Center in San Francisco. She is a Fellow of the Society for Clinical and Experimental Hypnosis and of the American Society of Clinical Hypnosis. She has received several awards for her writing, teaching, and clinical work, and is also the recipient of the Cornelia Wilbur Award for original contributions to the field of dissociation. She is a past editor of the* American Journal of Clinical Hypnosis. *She is the coauthor of* Healing the Divided Self: Clinical and Ericksonian Hypnotherapy for Post-Traumatic and Dissociative Conditions *and* Inner Strengths: Contemporary Psychotherapy and Hypnosis for Ego-Strengthening.

# Preface

Depression is one of the most common psychological disorders treated by family physicians, psychiatrists, and therapists. It is a heterogeneous biopsychosocial disorder, comprising multiple components. It is surprising that so little has been written on hypnotherapy in the treatment of depressive disorders. The little literature that exists consists of anecdotes, case studies, and a hodgepodge of techniques that do not clarify exactly how they are used to modify depression. Some clinicians say they use "dissociation" to treat depression; others use "forward projection." This reminds me of the therapist who says "I treat eating disorders with hypnosis" or "I treat eating disorders with solution-focused therapy." Although there may be some truth in these statements, the real truth is that we need multiple therapeutic approaches to treat eating disorder, because it is so complex a problem. Similarly, depression is a complex heterogeneous disorder, requiring multiple interventions. No one treatment universally works for every depressed patient. Another factor that might have impeded the development of a comprehensive hypnotherapy program for depression is the erroneous belief propagated by some well-known writers that hypnosis exacerbates suicidal behavior.

Two developments occurring in the field during the past 20 years are beginning to change the scene. First, Dr. Michael Yapko has written several books on the application of hypnotherapy as an adjunct treatment for depression (one component of a comprehensive approach). The second development relates to the cognitive revolution in psychotherapy. Cognitive behavior therapy (CBT), in over 80 randomized controlled trials, has been demonstrated to be a very effective treatment for depression. CBT also provides a theory of depression, and the treatment approach is very comprehensive, comprising cognitive and behavioral techniques. Nevertheless, not every depressed patient responds to CBT; a significant number of patients do not respond to CBT, and a large proportion of patients treated with CBT relapse. Several reviews and meta-analyses have demonstrated that when hypnotherapy is combined with CBT and other forms of psychotherapy, the effect size increases. My interest in writing this book was sparked by these findings and fueled by my own study that compared the effect of CBT with cognitive hypnotherapy (hypnotherapy combined with CBT) in a sample of 84 chronically depressed patients (see Chapter 5). The study clearly demonstrated that the effect size is increased when hypnotherapy is combined with CBT.

The purpose of this book is to serve as a manual for the use of cognitive hypnotherapy with depression. The treatment protocols, based on empirical evidence, are clearly described so that other clinicians can utilize them in their practice. However, the book should not be used simply as a manual; it can be utilized as a springboard for expanding and developing other treatment strategies. The book advocates for *evidence-based practice in psychology* (EBPP), which supersedes *empirically supported treatments* (ESTs). EBPP is a hybrid approach to psychotherapy that integrates efficacy with effectiveness. EBPP specifically integrates best available research with clinical expertise in the context of patient characteristics, culture, and preferences. EBPP promotes effective psychological practice and enhances public health by applying empirically supported principles of psychological assessment, case formulation, therapeutic relationship, and intervention. Because this book adopts the EBPP model, I chose to title it *Handbook of Cognitive Hypnotherapy for Depression: An Evidence-Based Approach*.

Because of its complexity, depression is not an easy disorder to treat, and therapists can become easily demoralized. Therefore, another goal of the book is to share my 25 years of clinical experience in treating depression; I hope some of the techniques described here empower therapists to take a fresh approach. The chapters on First Aid for Depression, Developing Antidepressive Pathways, Breaking Ruminative Patterns, and Mindfulness and Acceptance will hopefully provide some innovative and practical approaches for working with depression. The book also addresses the neglected area of relapse prevention; a whole chapter (Chapter 16) is devoted to illustrating how hypnotherapy can be effectively utilized to prevent relapse in depression.

The term *patient* is used throughout to emphasize the treatment aspects of clinical depression, although I recognize that some valid reasons exist for using the term *client* in many situations. I also use the term *hypnotherapy* for clinical hypnosis to emphasize its clinical applications, and the term *hypnosis* is restricted to the scientific or theoretical construct. Usages of these terms are not meant to provide new definitions.

I hope this volume will serve to stimulate future research and developments in the application of hypnosis in the management of clinical depression.

*Assen Alladin*

# Acknowledgments

There are many people I would like to thank for their continuing support and assistance with this project.

My son, Adam, who constantly inspired me by inquiring about the contents and my progress with the book. Farrah, my daughter, who stayed in the background, but who initially suggested that I should write the book. And my wife, Naseem, who kept reminding me that I should finish the project by the deadline.

Dr. Michael Yapko, who unselfishly shared his experience and wisdom in getting the work published. Dr. Claire Frederick, who provided encouragement and support to persevere with the project.

I would also like to thank Jim Arthurs, unit manager, and Dr. Michael King, psychology manager, from Foothills Medical Centre for providing encouragement and allowing me some time off to work on this project.

I also want to thank Charles Mitchell, publisher, medical practice division, from Lippincott Williams & Wilkins, for providing his support and recognizing the value of the book. Thanks are also due to Jenny Koleth, freelance developmental editor, for her support and guidance with the chapters. Finally, I would like to thank Stan Wakefield from Electronic & Database Publishing, Inc., who started the ball rolling 3 years ago.

# Current Perspective

# Current Theories and Treatment of Depression

**DEFINITION AND DESCRIPTION OF DEPRESSION**

Depression encompasses a wide range of clinical entities, from a mild mood disturbance commonly found in both normal and anxious persons to a serious, potentially lethal medical illness. Moreover, depression can be either a central or an associated feature of many types of mental disorders. Clinical depression can be defined as a condition characterized by a persistent and abnormal lowering of mood (feeling sad, blue, unhappy) and/or a loss of interest in usual activities, accompanied by a variety of characteristic signs and symptoms. The signs and symptoms of clinical depression are observed in five distinct, but related areas:

*Negative affect:* Characterized by low mood, loss of pleasure, and feelings of guilt, nervousness, irritability, and boredom.

*Negative cognitions:* Negative view of the self, the world and the future; indecisiveness, self-blame and feelings of worthlessness and hopelessness.

*Negative motivations:* Loss of interest, suicidal ideation, social withdrawal, and neglect of appearance and hygiene.

*Behavioral changes:* Reduction in activities or psychomotor retardation, and agitation.

*Vegetative changes:* Insomnia, loss of appetite and weight, reduced libido, vague aches and pains.

Since first described by Hippocrates as a medical illness, depression has undergone many transformations through the centuries. In the 1930s, Manfred Blueler classified depressive disorders under the term "affective" disorders. More recently, the revised fourth edition of the *Diagnostic and Statistical Manual (DSM-IV-TR),* published by the American Psychiatric Association (2000), replaced affective disorders by the term "mood" disorders in order to emphasize the gross deviation in mood. Although the *DSM-IV-TR* classification of mood disorders is not entirely satisfactory, it is the most widely used classification. Since no perfect system of classification exists, any classification of mood disorders is likely to be controversial. Because this book is confined to major depressive disorder (MDD), the terms depression, affective disorder, mood disorder, or unipolar depression are used interchangeably to denote nonbipolar depressions.

*DSM-IV-TR* divides mood disorders into *bipolar* and *depressive* disorders. Bipolar disorders are characterized by the presence of depressive symptoms and one or more episodes of *mania* (elevated mood, increased activity, and expansive and self-important ideas) or *hypomania* (mild mania). Depressive disorders are subdivided into major depressive disorder (MDD), dysthymic disorder (DD), and depressive disorder not otherwise specified (DDNOS). These disorders exclude a history of manic, mixed, or hypomanic episodes, and they should not be due to the physiological effects of substances of abuse, other medications, or toxins (First & Tasman, 2004).

### *DSM-IV-TR* Criteria for Major Depressive Disorder

The formal diagnosis of MDD is made when five of the following symptoms are present for at least 2 weeks (either depressed mood or loss of interest and pleasure must be one of the five symptoms):

1. Sad or depressed mood most of the day, nearly every day (or irritable mood in children or adolescents).
2. Significant loss of interest and pleasure in all or almost all activities.
3. Poor appetite and marked weight loss, or increased appetite and weight gain.
4. Insomnia or hypersomnia nearly every day.
5. Fatigue or lack of energy nearly every day.
6. Psychomotor agitation or retardation nearly every day.
7. Diminished ability to think or concentrate, or indecisiveness.
8. Feelings of worthlessness and guilt, and negative self-concept, self-reproach and self-blame.
9. Recurrent thoughts of death or suicide.

### *DSM-IV-TR* Criteria for Dysthymic Disorder

Dysthymic disorder (DD), previously known as depressive neurosis, is a chronic, mild-to-moderate form of clinical depression, prevalent for at least 2 years. Unlike MDD, DD has only one typical presentation and, because of its relatively constant course, there is some controversy whether dysthymia should be considered a specific disorder or a personality disorder (Arean & Chatav, 2003). The formal DSM-IV-TR diagnosis for DD is made when a person has been depressed most days, for most of the week for 2 years and presented two or more of these six symptoms: (i) poor appetite and overeating, (ii) insomnia or hypersomnia, (iii) low energy or fatigue, (iv) low self-esteem, (v) poor concentration or difficulty making decisions, and (vi) feelings of hopelessness. During the 2-year episode (1 year for children or adolescents), the symptoms of dysthymia must not be absent for more than 2 months at a time. Moreover, no major depressive episode must have been present during the first 2 years of the disturbance, and the symptoms must not be due to other nonaffective disorders such as schizophrenia or chronic medical conditions or to the direct physiological effects of a substance (including medication). In addition, the person must not have ever met criteria for manic episode, hypomanic episode, or cyclothymic disorder.

Approximately 25% of patients with depressive disorders present the diagnosis of *double depression* (Keller & Shapiro, 1982) or concurrent presence of both major depression and DD. This is a chronic condition marked by episodes of MDD in dysthymic patients. The course of double depression has two notable characteristics compared to MDD. First, patients with double depression recover more rapidly from episodes of major depression than do patients with MDD only (Boland & Keller, 2002). However, the recovery is not complete, but to a level of dysthymia. Second, patients with double depression are more likely to relapse than those patients with major depression alone.

### Depressive Disorder Not Otherwise Specified

Depressive disorder NOS (DDNOS) refers to a variety of conditions listed in *DSM-IV-TR* that do not meet formal criteria for MDD or DD. The conditions listed under this category include premenstrual dysphoric disorder, minor depressive disorder, recurrent brief depressive disorder, postpsychotic depressive disorder of schizophrenia, and depressive episode superimposed on delusional disorder or other psychotic disorder. It is important to note that DDNOS is associated with impairment in overall functioning and general health, and it affects 8% to 11% of the population (First & Tasman, 2004).

There has been considerable debate whether subtypes of depression should be classed as discrete illnesses or seen as dimensions of a single illness along a severity continuum (Arean & Chatav, 2003). However, as knowledge of depression advances, there is a strong movement toward considering both arguments in the diagnosis and treatment of depression. Since MDD has been most researched and understood, the rest of the chapter focuses on MDD when discussing the prevalence, course, etiology, and treatment of depression. Throughout the book, the words depression, mood disorder, or unipolar depression will be used to refer to MDD. However, the treatment techniques described are equally applicable to dysthymia and DDNOS.

## PREVALENCE AND COURSE OF DEPRESSION

Depression is among one of the most common psychiatric disorders treated by psychiatrists and psychotherapists, and approximately one half of all psychiatric admissions are depressed patients. Both American and British statistics suggest that the lifetime expectancy of developing unipolar depression is approximately 20% in women and 10% in men. The prevalence rate of depression is higher among people from the lower socioeconomic group; divorced and separated persons (Smith & Weissman, 1992); primary care outpatients with chronic disease (ranging from 9% to 20%; Barry, et al., 1998); and medical inpatients (15% to 36%; Feldman, et al., 1987). However, the majority of depressed people do not seek or receive treatment. The estimated percentages of severely depressed patients receiving treatment range from 20% to 33% worldwide (Kaplan & Sardock, 1981).

Apart from being one of the most commonly diagnosed psychological disorders, major depressive disorder is reported to be on the increase (World Health Organization, 1998). It is estimated that out of every 100 people, approximately 13 men and 21 women are likely to develop the disorder at some point in life (Kessler, et al., 1994), and approximately one third of the population may suffer from mild depression at some point in their lives (Paykel & Priest, 1992). In fact, the rate of major depression is so high that the World Health Organization (WHO) Global Burden of Disease Study ranked depression as the single most burdensome disease in the world, in terms of total disability adjusted life years among people during the middle years of life (Murray & Lopez, 1996). Major depression is also a very costly disorder in terms of lost productivity at work, industrial accidents, beds occupancy in hospitals, treatment, state benefits, and personal suffering. The disorder also adversely affects interpersonal relationships with spouses and children (Gotlib & Hammen, 2002), and the rate of divorce is higher among depressives than among nondepressed individuals (e.g., Wade & Cairney, 2000). The children of depressed parents are found to be at elevated risk of psychopathology (Gotlib & Goodman, 1999). According to WHO (1998), by 2020, clinical depression is likely to be second only to chronic heart disease as an international health burden, as measured by cause of death, disability, incapacity to work, and medical resources used.

Moreover, depression has significant impact on mortality. The link between depression and mortality is most noticeable in patients with cardiovascular disease. A twofold elevated risk of mortality is noted in patients with depression recovering from myocardial infarction (Frasure, Smith, Lesperance, & Talajic, 1995). Similarly, the mortality rate for depressive older adults residing in nursing homes is twice of those without depression (Rovner, 1993). Furthermore, about 15% of patients suffering from primary mood disorder ultimately take their own lives (Stolberg, Clark, & Bongar, 2002).

A *major depressive episode* is the most common form of depression diagnosed in clinical practice. If two or more major depressive episodes occur, separated by a period of at least 2 months, during which the individual was not depressed, *major depressive disorder, recurrence*, is diagnosed. Approximately 60% of people who have a major depressive episode will have a second episode. Among those who have experienced two episodes, 70% will have a third, and among those who have had three episodes, 90% will have a fourth (American Psychiatric Association, 2000). Recurrence is very important in predicting the future course of the disorder, as well as in choosing appropriate treatments. As many as 85% of single-episode cases later experience a second episode. The median lifetime number of major depressive episodes is four, and 25% of depressed patients experience six or more episodes (Angst & Preizig, 1996). Depression therefore is considered to be a chronic condition that waxes and wanes over time but seldom disappears (Solomon, et al., 2000). The median duration of recurrent depression is 5 months. Episodes of MDD are often triggered by severe psychosocial stressors, such as the death of a loved one or divorce. Studies indicate, however, that psychosocial stressors play a more significant role in the precipitation of the first or second episodes than in the onset of subsequent episodes (American Psychiatric Association, 2000).

Over 50% of depressed patients have their first episode of depression before the age of 40. An untreated episode of depression may last 6 to 13 months, whereas most treated episodes last about 3 months. Approximately 50% to 85% of patients have a second depressive episode within the next 4 to 6 months. The risk of recurrence is usually increased by coexisting dysthymia, alcohol or drug abuse, anxiety symptoms, older age at onset, and a history of more than one previous depressive episode. Approximately 50% of all depressed patients recover completely, but in 20% to 35% of cases, a chronic course ensues, with considerable residual symptomatic and social impairment (*DSM-IV-TR,* 2000).

In trying to define the course of major depressive disorder, researchers have come to realize that depression is a heterogeneous disorder, with many possible courses. Moreover, people with the same diagnosis may vary greatly from one another. For example, some depressed patients may be diagnosed as having psychotic features, such as delusions and hallucinations. Such distinction among unipolar depressives is important because it has implications both for treating and recognizing the severity of the illness. It has been proved that depressed patients with delusions do not generally respond well to antidepressants, but show better response when an antipsychotic drug is combined with the antidepressant. It is also known that depression with psychotic features tends to be more severe than depression without delusions, and it involves more social impairment and less time between episodes (Coryell, et al., 1996).

Moreover, depression co-occurs with other disorders, both medical and psychiatric. Kessler (2002), from his review of the epidemiology of depression, concludes that comorbidity is the norm among people with depression. For example, the Epidemiologic Catchment Area Study (Robins & Regier, 1991) found that 75% of respondents with lifetime depressive disorder also met criteria for at least one of the other DSM-III disorders assessed in that survey. Anxiety is the most frequent comorbid condition with depression. Approximately 50% to 76% of depressed patients experience anxiety (Dozois & Westra, 2004). In fact, considerable symptom overlap occurs between these two conditions. The presence of poor concentration, irritability, hypervigilance, fatigue, guilt, memory loss, sleep difficulties, and worry may suggest a diagnosis of either disorder. The symptom overlap between the two conditions may be indicative of similar neurobiologic correlates. At a psychologic level, it seems reasonable to assume that depression can result from the demoralization caused by anxiety, for example in a case of an agoraphobic who becomes withdrawn because of the fear of going out. Conversely, a person with depression may become anxious due to worry about being unable to hold gainful employment. Although there is an apparent overlap between anxiety and depression, it is common clinical practice to focus on treating one disorder at a time. Lack of an integrated approach to treatment may mean that a patient is treated only for depression while still suffering from anxiety. One of the rationales for combining hypnosis with cognitive behavior therapy, as described in this book, is to address symptoms of anxiety.

## THEORIES OF DEPRESSION

Despite the well-known fact that many types of depression exist, each involving multiple factors in the genesis of the disorders, researchers have expended a great deal of energy finding a single cause of depression. Some of the well-known biological and psychological theories of depression are briefly and selectively reviewed here to underline the limitation of searching for a single cause of depression. The cognitive theory of depression is described in greater details in the next chapter, because it forms part of the integrated model of depression (Cognitive-Dissociative Model of Depression) described in Chapter 4.

## Biological Theories

The biological theories of depression have mainly focused on genetic predisposition, neurochemistry, the neuroendocrine system, and structural changes in the brain.

Research on the role of genetic transmission in depression has focused on family, twin, and adoption studies. The genetic information available indicates that unipolar depression clusters in first-degree relatives of individuals with depression. But this observation does not address the issue of whether the familial aggregation is due to genetic or familial environmental factors. As multiple psychosocial risk factors such as gender, early parental loss, parental separation, rearing patterns, trauma and abuse, personality factors, prior major depression, low social class, and stressful recent life events are associated with depression (Kendler, et al., 1993), it would appear that environmental risk factors not shared by relatives are clearly important in the etiology of depression. Although specific life events can trigger the initial episode of depression, it is not known whether they have a similar impact on the subsequent precipitation of depressive episodes. Post (1992) argues that, while adverse life events are associated with the initial or second episode of depression, subsequent recurrent episodes are associated with neurobiological factors. Post further asserts that sensitization to stressors and episodes may become encoded at the level of gene expression, underscoring the role of neurobiological factors in the progression of depressive illness. An individual's social support and effective treatment can, however, protect the individual from the vulnerability of recurrent episodes (First & Tasman, 2004).

Since the advent of effective antidepressant drugs in the 1950s, the past 40 years have seen active research into the biological determinants of depression. From this area of research, several biochemical theories of depression have been proposed, including the hypotheses that (a) a deficiency of important neurotransmitters (such as norepinephrine and serotonin) occurs in certain areas of the brain; (b) an abnormality is present in the functioning of the neuroendocrine system that regulates hormonal secretion and other important biological activities; and (c) some structural changes occur in the brains of depressed individuals.

It was initially believed that depression was caused, in part, by lack of the neurotransmitters norepinephrine and serotonin. Recent studies have challenged this simple paradigm, and it is now known that it is the *dysregulation* rather than the *deficiency* of these neurotransmitters that cause depression (Moore & Bona, 2001). Recently, researchers have focused on the postsynaptic effects of antidepressants and are beginning to develop theories of depression that implicate postsynaptic mechanisms (Veenstra-VanderWeele, Anderson, & Cook, 2000). The neurotransmitter theory of depression, although important, provides only a partial picture of the biological origin of depression. Moreover, abnormalities in neurotransmitter regulation do not always lead to depression.

The contribution of endocrine system alterations in depression has been studied extensively. Both hypothyroidism and hyper-cortisolism may result in depression. Although some depressed patients may have a thyroid dysfunction, the role of thyroid in depression is unclear (First & Tasman, 2004). The evidence for the role of the hypothalamic-pituitary-adrenocortical axis (HPA) in depression is much stronger. Various findings support the hy-pothesis that an overabundance of cortisol (an adrenocortical hormone) is present in the systems of depressed patients, re-sulting from oversecretion of thyrotropin-releasing hormone by the hypothalamus (Garbutt, et al., 1994). Because the HPA axis is interconnected with multiple neurotransmitters such as 5-hydroxytryptamine (5HT), norepinephrine (NE), (acetylcholine) Ach, and gamma-aminobutyric acid (GABA), neuroendocrinology provides a more complete understanding of the biological causes of depression. However, the complex interrelation and inter-dependence of neurochemical systems involving critical neuro-transmitters, synaptic regulation, nerve cell mediation and mod-ulation, neuropeptides, and neuroendocrine systems are poorly understood (First & Tasman, 2004). Moreover, biochemical re-search is beginning to indicate that depressed patients may form biological subtypes, although a group of patients may appear clinically similar (Duman, Heninger, & Nestler, 1997). It is also known that individuals without any biochemical aberration may exhibit erratic regulation of the neurotransmitters in response to exogenous factors, such as bereavement or losing one's job. How-ever, this should not underestimate the considerable progress of biochemical research in the somatic treatment of depression.

Physiological changes in the brain structures of depressed in-dividuals provide support for structural changes in the brains of people with depression. Sheline (2000) demonstrated that early-onset depression and late-onset depression are associated with different loci of changes in the brain. Brain changes in early-onset depression were localized in the hippocampus, amygdala, caudate nucleus, putamen, and frontal cortex, whereas late-onset depression was noted to frequently occur with comorbid physical illnesses that often affect brain structures involved in emotion regulation. Arean and Chatav (2003) argue that, because these physical changes can occur during stress and are closely associ-ated with depression, the physiological changes in brain structure hypothesis provides a more comprehensive picture and explana-tion of the causes of depression.

## Psychological Theories

As noted earlier, some data support the biological etiology of de-pression. Does this mean that psychological theories are irrele-vant? In fact, all the major psychological theories of psychopathol-ogy assert that behavioral disorders are mediated by biological processes and bodily changes. Similarly, most biological psychi-atrists consider depression to result from the disruption of bio-logical rhythms caused by psychosocial stressors. For example, Ehlers, et al. (1988) have proposed the *social zeitgebers theory* to explain the link between biological and psychosocial factors in the causation of depression. The social zeitgebers theory sug-gests that social relationships, interpersonal continuity, and work tasks entrain the biological rhythms (First & Tasman, 2004). Biological rhythms that maintain homeostasis are affected by disruption of the social rhythms caused by such psychosocial stressor as loss of a relationship. The biological disruption leads to changes in such neurobiological processes as neurotransmitter function, neuroendocrine regulation, and oscillation of the circadian rhythms. Therefore, biological and psychological factors should not be considered incompatible, but complementary to each other.

The psychodynamic, behavioral, learned helplessness and hopelessness, and interpersonal theories of depression are briefly described to highlight the role of psychological factors in the etiology of depression. The cognitive theory of depression is described in greater detail in Chapter 2, because the cognitive-dissociative conceptualization of depression presented in Chapter 4 and the cognitive therapy described later in the book are largely derived from the cognitive theory of depression.

## Psychodynamic Theories

Psychodynamic theories of depression are complex and varied, although they all emphasize unconscious mental processes and psychic conflict of wishes and feelings in the genesis of clinical depression. Some of the well-known psychodynamic postulates are listed below:

1. Real or symbolic loss of a loved object is at the root of clinical depression (Abraham, 1911; Freud, 1917).
2. Depression results from psychic conflict between love and hate (Abraham, 1911; Freud, 1917).
3. Depression results from psychic conflict between rage and guilt (Rado, 1951).
4. Loss of self-esteem is of central importance in depressive disorders (Bibring, 1953).
5. Depression results from an unconscious conflict between ideals and self-perception (Bibring, 1953).
6. Depression results from unsuccessful efforts to cope with unpleasant emotions (Brenner, 1979).
7. Depression results from premature and unsubstituted loss of the mother–infant attachment bond (Bowlby, 1977).

Although unconscious mental processes may influence the development and course of depression in some individuals, psychodynamic theories of depression are lacking because (i) the above postulates are not applicable to all types of depression; (ii) there is no evidence that low self-esteem is more common in people who develop depression; (iii) in some depressed patients, anger is directed toward people or objects other than the self (Weissman, Klerman, & Paykel, 1971); (iv) some studies have found that depression is not associated with parental death, divorce, broken engagements, and similar losses of a significant relationship (Malmquist, 1970; Watts & Nicoli, 1979); and (v) clinical and epidemiologic studies do not firmly support the hypothesis that separation during childhood predisposes to adult depression.

However, some personality factors might be associated with the onset and maintenance of depression. Beck (1983) proposed that depression is associated with two personality styles: *sociotropy* and *autonomy*. Sociotropic individuals are socially driven—they are dependent on others, and eager to please others, avoid disapproval, and avoid separation. Autonomy individuals are achievement-orientated. They are self-critical, goal-driven, desire solitude, and seek freedom. Research using the revised Sociotropy-Autonomy Scale by Clark, et al. (1995) has shown that sociotropy is linked with depression, while autonomy is not consistently correlated with depression. Similarly Blatt (1974, 1995) has suggested that introjective and anaclitic personality styles are associated with vulnerability to depression. While the *introjective orientation* involves excessive levels of self-criticism, the *anaclitic orientation* involves excessive levels of dependency on others. Extensive research with the Depressive Experiences Questionnaire (DEQ), developed by Blatt (1974, 1995) to measure self-criticism and dependency, has shown a strong association between self-criticism and depression, but a weaker link between dependency and depression (Mongrain & Zuroff, 1994). Moreover, the concept of self-criticism is closely linked with perfectionism (Blatt, 1995). Several studies found elevated levels of socially prescribed perfectionism, excessive concern over mistakes, and self-criticism among depressed patients (Enns & Cox, 1999). Moreover, perfectionism has been found to be linked with chronic symptoms of unipolar and bipolar depression (Hewitt, Flett, Ediger, Norton, & Flynn, 1998). However, personality factors on their own may not produce depressive symptoms. The *congruency hypothesis* (Wildes, Harkness, & Simons, 2002) has been proposed to explain that personality factors interact with psychosocial stressors to produce symptoms. The congruency hypothesis has received mixed support.

## Learned Helplessness and Hopelessness

Drawing on data from animal studies, Seligman (1975) proposed the "learned helplessness" model of depression. The model asserts that repeated exposure to uncontrollable events leads to motivational, affective, and cognitive deficits. Consequently, depressed persons fail to accurately perceive a response–outcome contingency when outcomes are contingent upon their own performance. Using an animal model, Seligman posited learned uncontrollability (faulty learning) to be the key determination of depression; that is, depression develops under conditions of uncontrollable failure and elicits reinforcement for repeated failure.

This model was later reformulated to include attributional style, and the studies were carried out using human subjects. Abramson, Seligman, and Teasdale (1978) suggested that expectations of future uncontrollability, rather than faulty learning, are critical in determining the symptoms of helplessness and their consequent effect on self-esteem, mood, motivation, and cognition (learning)—the four key components of clinical depression. The theory suggests that people become depressed when they attribute negative life events to *stable* ("I'm weird, abnormal"), *global* ("I can never do anything right"), and *internal* characteristics ("I'm stupid") causes. The theory considers an individual prone to depression as having a depressive attributional style and a tendency to attribute bad outcomes to personal stable faults of character. Recently, this theory too has been reformulated to include the concept of *hopelessness* (Abramson, Metalsky, Alloy, 1989). Some forms of depression (hopelessness depressions) are now regarded as caused by a state of hopelessness—an expectation that desirable outcomes will not occur or that undesirable ones will occur, and that the person has no resources available to change this situation. As in the attributional theory, negative life events (stressors) are seen as interacting with diatheses to yield a state of hopelessness. In addition to the attributional pattern diathesis, this theory encompasses two additional diatheses: Low self-esteem and the tendency to infer that negative life events will have severe negative consequences. The hopelessness theory of depression was supported by several studies. For example, Lewinshon, et al. (1974) found that a patient's attributional style and low self-esteem predicted the onset of depression in adolescents. According to Alloy, et al. (1990), expectation of helplessness creates anxiety. Because 70% to 76% of depressed patients have comorbid anxiety (Dozois & Westra, 2004), the advantage of the hopelessness theory over other theories is that it can directly explain anxiety.

Although these theories are promising, and have generated extensive research and theorizing about depression, some difficulties arise in extrapolating the findings to clinical depression. Because most human studies have relied on the experimental induction of depression in normal or mildly depressed subjects, the findings cannot be easily generalized to clinical depression. Moreover, some of the studies have failed to distinguish between the symptoms of depression and *depressive syndrome* (a group of symptoms occurring together, constituting a recognizable condition).

## Behavioral Theory of Depression

Lewinshon and colleagues (1974, 1986) proposed that depression develops when individuals stop receiving adequate positive reinforcement from their environments, while simultaneously experiencing "punishing" experiences. Lewinshon suggests three general reasons for the development of such reinforcement patterns: (i) the individual's environment may actually contain few positive elements (e.g., living in an isolated area while craving for many friendships), (ii) an individual may lack social skills to obtain positive results or cope with negative consequences, and (iii) an individual may interpret events in a way that minimizes the positive and accentuates the negative. According to Lewinshon, when behavior decreases due to nonreinforcement, the other symptoms of depression, such as low energy and low self-esteem, will follow more or less automatically. In general, research has provided some support for the behavioral theory of depression (e.g., Rehm & Tyndall, 1993). However, the strictly behavioral approach to understanding the complexity of depression has been seen as rather simple and, consequently, the strictly behavioral approach to understanding and treating depression has been replaced by a cognitive–behavioral hybrid (see Chapter 2).

## Interpersonal Theory of Depression

The interpersonal theories of depression focus on a person's close relationships and their roles in those relationships (Klerman, et al., 1984). Depression is seen to result from disturbances in these roles. These disturbances may be recent or rooted in long-standing patterns of interactions. The theory draws from Bowlby's (1982) attachment theory, which argues that children who do not experience their caregivers as reliable, responsive, and warm develop an insecure attachment to these caregivers, which sets the stage for all future relationships. These problematic relationships are internalized as negative working models of others and of the self in relation to others. Children with insecure attachments develop *contingencies of self-worth* (Kuiper & Olinger, 1986), which are expectations that they must be or do certain things in order to win the approval of others. As long as the individual meets the internalized contingencies of self-worth, positive self-esteem and a nondepressed state are maintained; but if the contingencies are not met, the person plunges into depression. Contingencies of self-worth are similar to the dysfunctional beliefs described by cognitive theorists (see Chapter 2), except that the interpersonal theorists emphasize that dysfunctional beliefs originate from insecure attachment in childhood.

The interpersonal theories of depression have been supported in several studies. For example, Roberts, Gotlib, and Kassel (1996), in a longitudinal study of college students, demonstrated that those with an anxious, insecure attachment style had more dysfunctional negative beliefs and subsequently lower self-esteem and more depressive symptoms. The main weakness of the interpersonal models of depression is that the focus of most research has been on the evaluation of the therapy based on the model, rather than on the various interpersonal theories.

## CURRENT TREATMENTS

Just as there are many theories of depression, so there are many approaches to treatment. Each approach to treatment is applied in a manner that is consistent with its associated theory of etiology. However, none of the treatment approaches is effective with every depressed patient. Currently, the main available treatment for clinical depression is pharmacotherapy, specifically the use of various antidepressant medications such as tricyclics, monoamine oxidase inhibitors (MAOIs), and selective serotonergic reuptake inhibitors (SSRIs). Medication is most effective in reducing signs and symptoms during the acute phase of the illness.

Tricyclic antidepressant drugs such as *imipramine* (Tofranil) and *amitriptyline* (Elavil) are widely used for the treatment of depression, and they have been around since the 1960s. Although these drugs reduce acute symptoms in about 60% of depressed patients (Nemeroff, 2000), they can take about 4 to 8 weeks to work (Fava & Rosenbaum, 1995) and, during this time, many patients may feel worse and may develop a number of side effects such as blurred vision, dry mouth, constipation, difficulty urinating, drowsiness, weight gain, and possible sexual dysfunction. For this reason, about 40% of these patients may stop the medication, believing that the cure may be worse than the illness (Barlow & Durand, 2005). Moreover, tricyclics may be lethal if taken in excessive doses. For these reasons, physicians have been wary of using tricyclics in depressed patients, especially in those who may have suicidal thoughts. However, with careful management, many side effects may disappear.

Monoamine oxidase inhibitors (MAOIs) have also been used to treat depression, and they seem to be as effective as or slightly more effective than tricyclics (American Psychiatric Association, 2000). They have been less popular because of two potentially serious consequences. First, eating foods and drinking beverages containing tyramine (e.g., cheese, red wine, or beer) can lead to severe hypertensive episodes and, occasionally, even death. Second, other daily drugs such as cold medication can interact with MAOIs to produce dangerous and even fatal consequences. For these reasons, MAOIs are used only when other antidepressant medications do not work.

During the past 20 years, a second generation of antidepressants, known as selective serotonin reuptake inhibitors (SSRIs) have become extremely popular in the treatment of depression. The best-known SSRI is *fluoxetine* (Prozac), which was initially hailed as a breakthrough drug. These drugs are similar in structure to the tricyclics, but they work more selectively to affect serotonin. Although the SSRIs do not work better than tricyclics and MAOIs, they can produce improvement within a couple of weeks, and they produce less severe side effects. Moreover, these drugs are not fatal in overdose, and they appear to help with a range of disorders including anxiety, binge eating, and premenstrual symptoms (Pearlstein, et al., 1997). Some reports appearing in the press suggest that Prozac might lead to suicidal preoccupation, paranoid reactions, and occasionally, violence (e.g., Teicher, Glod, & Cole, 1990). These reports have not been substantiated by evidence. In fact, Fava and Rosenbaum (1991) found that the risks of suicide with Prozac were no greater than with any other antidepressant, and Olfson, et al. (2003), from a large community survey, found a slightly, but significant, decrease in suicide among adolescents taking SSRIs compared to depressed adolescents not taking SSRIs.

During the past decade, a number of other drugs, such as mirtazapine (Remeron), nefazodone (Serzone), venlafaxine (Effexor), and bupropion (Wellbutrin), have also been introduced. These drugs are often used in conjunction with SSRIs. Although a variety of antidepressants is available, there are no consistent rules for determining which of the antidepressants to use first. In clinical practice, the choice of a specific antidepressant is determined by the given clinical situation, history of response to medications, and co-occurring mental disorders. Often, several antidepressants are used, or an antidepressant is augmented by other drugs (e.g., lithium carbonate), before finding a drug regimen that work well and with tolerable side effects. Antidepressant medications have relieved severe depression and undoubtedly prevented suicide in tens of thousands of patients around the world. Although antidepressant medications are readily available and generally effective in reducing severe symptoms of depression, many people refuse or are not eligible to take them. Some people are wary of the long-term side effects, and some women of childbearing age refuse to take them for fear of damaging the fetus if they happen to conceive while taking antidepressants. Moreover, 40% to 50% of patients do not respond adequately to these drugs, and a substantial number of the remainder is left with residual symptoms of depression (Barlow & Durand, 2005). Several follow-up studies (Belsher & Costello, 1988; Paykel, et al., 1999; Rafanelli, Park & Fava, 1999) found that approximately 50% of depressed patients who are in remission or recovered from depression relapse following the discontinuation of either tricyclic medication or SSRIs.

Electroconvulsive therapy (ECT) is often given to patients with severe or psychotic depression who don't respond to drug therapies. ECT is known to relieve depression in 50% to 60% of depressed patients (Fink, 2001), and it is particularly useful in older adults who lack self-care or have significant weight loss (First & Tasman, 2004). ECT, however, remains a controversial treatment for several reasons: (i) it causes transitory cognitive and memory impairments, (ii) the idea of passing electrical current through a person's brain appears primitive, and (iii) it is still not known how ECT works.

Although antidepressant medications and ECT work well for many depressed persons, they do not alleviate the problems that might have caused the depression in the first place. Pills cannot improve the loss or grief, bad marriages, unhappy work situations, family conflicts, residual interpersonal disputes, and ongoing social deficits that precede depression. For these reasons, many depressed people benefit from psychotherapies designed to help them cope with the difficult life circumstances or personality vulnerabilities that put them at risk for depression. Psychotherapy is therefore recommended as an adjunct to pharmacotherapy or as an alternative effective treatment for mild to moderate depressives. Psychotherapy in addition to medication also reduces relapse rate and increases compliance to medication. Psychotherapy is also recommended for depressed patients with medical conditions (such as pregnancy and some heart problems) that preclude the use of medications.

Although behavioral, interpersonal, and psychodynamic approaches to treating depression are reported, cognitive therapy is considered to be the most effective and widely used psychological treatment for unipolar depression (reviewed in the next chapter). The behavioral approach to treatment attempts to increase the frequency of the patient's positively reinforcing interactions with the environment and to decrease the number of negative interactions. Patient may also be taught social and/or assertive skills. The goals of the interpersonal approach to treatment are twofold: (i) through education, depressive symptoms are reduced and self-esteem improved and, (ii) the patient is helped to develop more effective strategies for dealing with social and interpersonal relations. The psychodynamic approach to treatment aims to promote insight into the patient's depressogenic patterns and help the patient to resolve dependency, defenses, suppressed anger, and other painful feelings. Some of these approaches are incorporated in the comprehensive approach to treatment described in Part III of the book.

## SUMMARY

Depression is a heterogeneous disorder. None of the theories reviewed provides an adequate explanation for all the symptoms and subtypes of depression. The psychological theories have mainly focused on behavioral and cognitive changes, whereas the biological models have mainly concentrated on neurotransmitters and neuroendocrine activities. Since depression is generally regarded as a psychobiological disorder, it is intriguing that few studies have addressed the interrelationship between psychological and biological dysfunction. As regards treatment, although antidepressant medication, ECT, and some psychological therapies seem to be effective with clinical depression, a large proportion of chronic and resistant cases do not seem to respond to any of these treatments. Alternative treatments for these nonresponders are urgently needed. The comprehensive treatment approach described later in the book provides such an alternative. Moreover, a large number of depressed patients who recover from the acute depressive episode tend to relapse. Keller, et al. (1983) followed 141 successfully treated depressives for 13 months and found that 43 (30.5%) relapsed after having been well for at least 8 weeks. A more recent study by Paykel, et al. (1995) found that at least 50% of patients who recover from an initial episode of depression will have at least one subsequent depressive episode, and those patients with a history of two or more past episodes will have a 70% to 80% likelihood of recurrence in their lives (Consensus Developmental Panel, 1985). These findings led Judd (1997) to conclude that unipolar depression is a chronic, lifelong illness, with over 80% of risk for repeated episodes. These findings indicate the need for maintenance therapy. Chapter 16 describes several psychological strategies for preventing recurrence and relapse of depression.

## REFERENCES

Abraham, K. (1911). Notes on the psychoanalytic investigation and treatment of manic-depressive insanity and allied conditions. In K. Abraham (Ed.), *Selected Papers on Psychoanalysis*, London: Hogarth Press.

Abramson, L.Y., Metalsky, G.I., & Alloy, L.B. (1989). Hopelessness depression: A theory based subtype of depression. *Psychological Review*, 96, 358–372.

Abramson, L.Y., Seligman, M.E.P., & Teasdale, J.D. (1978). Learned-helplessness in humans: Critique and reformulation. *Journal of Abnormal Psychology*, 87, 49–74.

Alloy, L.B., Kelly, K.A., Mineka, S., & Clements, C.M. (1990). Co-morbidity in anxiety and depressive disorders: A helplessness/hopelessness perspective. In J.D. Maser & C.R. Cloninger (Eds.), *Comorbidity in anxiety and mood disorders*. Washington, DC: American Psychiatric Press.

American Psychiatric Association (2000). *Diagnostic and Statistical Manual of Mental Disorders*, 4th ed., Text Rev. Washington, DC: American Psychiatric Press.

Angst, J., & Preizig, M. (1996). Course of a clinical cohort of unipolar, bipolar and schizoaffective patients: Results of a prospective study from 1959 to 1985. *Schweizer Archiv fur Neurologie und Psychiatrie*, 146, 1–16.

Arean, P.A., & Chatav, Y. (2003). Mood disorders: Depressive disorders. In M. Hersen & S.M. Turner (Eds.), *Adult Psychopathology and Diagnosis* (pp. 286–312). New Jersey: John Wiley & Sons, Inc.

Barlow, D.H., & Durand, V.M. (2005). *Abnormal Psychology: An Integrative Approach*. Boston: Thomson Wadsworth.

Barry, K.L., Fleming, M.F., Manwell, L.B., Copeland, L.A., & Appel, S. (1998). Prevalence and factors associated with current and lifetime depression in older adult primary care patients. *Family Medicine*, 30, 366–371.

Beck, A.T. (1983). Cognitive therapy of depression: New approaches. In P. Clayton & J. Barrett (Eds.), *Treatment of Depression: Old and New Approaches* (pp. 265–290). New York: Raven Press.

Belsher, G., & Costello, C.G. (1988). Relapse after recovery from unipolar depression: A critical review. *Psychological Bulletin*, 104, 84–96.

Bibring, E. (1953). The mechanism of depression. In P. Greenacre (Ed.), *Affective Disorders*. New York: International Universities Press.

Blatt, S.J. (1974). Levels of object representation in anaclitic and introjective depression. *Psychoanalytic Study of the Child*, 29, 107–157.

Blatt, S.J. (1995). The destructiveness of perfectionism: Implications for the treatment of depression. *American Psychologist*, 50, 1003–1020.

Boland, R.J., & Keller, M.B. (2002). Course and outcome of depression. In I.H. Gotlib & C.L. Hammen (Eds.), *Handbook of Depression* (pp. 43–60). New York: Guilford Press.

Bowlby, J. (1977). The making and breaking of affectional bonds: I. Aetiology and psychopathology in the light of attachment theory. *British Journal of Psychiatry*, 130, 201–210.

Bowlby, J. (1982). *Attachment and Loss* (2nd ed.). New York: Basic Books.

Brenner, C. (1979). Depressive affect, anxiety, and psychic conflict in the phallic-oedipal phase. *Psychoanalytic Quarterly*, 48, 177–197.

Clark, D.A., Steer, R.A., Beck, A.T., & Ross, L. (1995). Psychometric characteristics of revised sociotropy and autonomy scales in college students. *Behavior Research and Therapy*, 33, 325–334.

Consensus Development Panel. (1985). NIMH/NIH consensus development conference statement: Mood disorders – Pharmacologic prevention of recurrence. *American Journal of Psychiatry*, 142, 469–476.

Coryell, W., Leon, A., Winokur, G., Endicott, J., Keller, M., Akiskal, H.S., & Solomon, D. (1996). Importance of psychotic features to long-term course in major depressive disorder. *American Journal of Psychiatry*, 153, 483–489.

Dozois, D.J.A., & Westra, H.A. (2004). The nature of anxiety and depression: Implications for prevention. In D.J.A. Dozois & K.S. Dobson (Eds.), *The Prevention of Anxiety and Depression: Theory, Research, and Practice* (pp. 43–71). Washington, DC: American Psychological Association.

Duman, S., Heninger, G.R., & Nestler, E.J. (1997). A molecular and cellular theory of depression. *Archives of General Psychiatry*, 54, 597–606.

Ehlers, C.L., Frank, E., & Kupfer, D.J. (1988). Social zeitgebers and biological rhythms: A unified approach to understanding the etiology of depression. *Archives of General Psychiatry*, 45, 948–952.

Enns, M.W., & Cox, B.J. (1999). Perfectionism and depressive symptom severity in major depressive disorder. *Behavior Therapy and Research*, 37, 783–794.

Fava, M., & Rosenbaum, J.F. (1991). Suicidality and fluoxetine: Is there a relationship? *Journal of Clinical Psychiatry*, 52(3), 108–111.

Fava, M., & Rosenbaum, J.F. (1995). Pharmacotherapy and somatic therapies. In E.E. Beckham & W.R. Leber (Eds.), *Handbook of Depression* (2nd ed., pp. 280–301). New York: Guilford Press.

Feldman, E., Mayou, R., Hawton, K., Ardern, M., & Smith, E.B. (1987). Psychiatric disorder in medical inpatients. *Quarterly Journal of Medicine*, 63, 405–412.

Fink, M. (2001). Convulsive therapy: A review of the first 55 years. *Journal of Affective Disorders*, 63, 1–15.

First, M.B., & Tasman, A. (2004). *DSM-IV-TR Mental Disorders: Diagnosis, Etiology, and Treatment*. Chichester, West Sussex: John Wiley & Sons, Ltd.

Frasure-Smith, N., Lesperance, F., & Talajic, M. (1995). The impact of negative emotions on prognosis following myocardial infarction: Is it more than depression? *Health Psychology*, 14, 388–398.

Freud, S. (1917). Mourning and melancholia. In *The Standard Edition of the Complete Psychological Works,* Vol. 14. London: Hogarth Press.

Garbutt, J.C., Mayo, J.P., Little, K.Y., Gillette, G.M., Mason, G.A., et al. (1994). Dose-response studies with protirelin. *Archives of General Psychiatry*, 51, 875–883.

Gotlib, I.H., & Goodman, S.H. (1999). Children of parents with depression. In W.K. Silverman & T.H. Ollendick (Eds.), *Developmental Issues in the Clinical Treatment of Children* (pp. 415–432). Boston: Allyn & Bacon.

Gotlib, I.H., & Hammen, C.L. (2002). Introduction. In I.H. Gotlib & C.L. Hammen (Eds.), *Handbook of Depression* (pp. 1–20). New York: Guilford Press.

Hewitt, P.L., Flett, G.L., Ediger, E., Norton, G.R., & Flynn, C.A. (1998). Perfectionism in chronic and state symptom of depression. *Canadian Journal of Behavioral Science*, 30, 234–242.

Judd, L.L. (1997). The clinical course of unipolar major depressive disorders. *Archives of General Psychiatry*, 54, 989–991.

Kaplan, H.I., & Sadock, B.J. (1981). *Modern Synopsis of Comprehensive Textbook of Psychiatry*, 3rd ed. Baltimore: Williams & Wilkins.

Keller, M.B., Lavori, P.W., Lewis, C.E., & Klerman, G.L. (1983). Predictors of relapse in major depressive disorder. *Journal of the American Medical Association*, 250, 3299–3304.

Keller, M., & Shapiro, R.W. (1982). "Double depression": Superimposition of acute depressive episodes on chronic depressive disorders. *American Journal of Psychiatry*, 139, 438–442.

Kendler, K.S., Neale, M.C., Kessler, R.C., Heath, A.C., & Eaves, L.J. (1993). A test of the equal-environment assumption in twin studies of psychiatric illness. *Behavior Genetics*, 23, 21–28.

Kessler, R.C. (2002). Epidemiology of depression. In I.H. Gotlib & C.C. Hammen (Eds.), *Handbook of Depression* (pp. 23–42). New York: Guilford Press.

Kessler, R.C., McGongale, K.A., Zhao, S., Nelson, C.B., Hughes, M., Eshleman, S., et al. (1994). Lifetime and 12-month prevalence of DSM-III-R psychiatric disorders in the United States: Results from the National Comorbidity Survey. *Archives of General Psychiatry*, 51, 8–19.

Klerman, G.L., Weissman, M.M., Rounsaville, B., & Chevron, E. (1984). *Interpersonal Psychotherapy of Depression*. New York: Basic Books.

Kuiper, N.A., & Olinger, L.J. (1986). Dysfunctional attitudes and a self-worth contingency model of depression. *Advances in Cognitive-Behavioral Research & Therapy*, 5, 115–142.

Lewinshon, P.M. (1974). A behavioral approach to depression. In R.J. Friedman & M.M. Katz (Eds.), *The Psychology of Depression: Contemporary Theory and Research*. Washington, DC: Winston-Wiley.

Lewinshon, P.M., Munoz, R.F., Youngren, M.A., & Zeiss, A.M. (1986). *Control Your Depression*. Engelwood Cliffs, NJ: Prentice Hall.

Malmquist, C.P. (1970). Depression and object loss in psychiatric admissions. *American Journal of Psychiatry*, 126, 1782–1787.

Mongrain, M., & Zuroff, D.C. (1994). Ambivalence over emotional expression and negative life events: Mediators for depression in dependent and self-critical individuals. *Personality and Individual Differences*, 16, 447–458.

Moore, J.D., & Bona, J.R. (2001). Depression and dysthymia. *Medical Clinics of North America*, 85(3), 631–644.

Murray, C.J.L., & Lopez, A.D. (Eds.). (1996). *The Global Burden of Disease: A Comprehensive Assessment of Mortality and Disability from Diseases, Injuries, and Risk Factors in 1990 and Projected to 2020*. Cambridge, MA: Harvard University Press.

Nemeroff, C.B. (2000). An ever-increasing pharmacopoeia for the management of patients with bipolar disorder. *Journal of Clinical Psychiatry*, 61(Suppl. 13), 19–25.

Olfson, M., Shaffer, D., Marcus, S.C., & Greenberg, T. (2003). Relationship between antidepressant medication treatment and suicide in adolescents. *Archives of General Psychiatry*, 60, 978–982.

Paykel, E.S., & Priest, R.G. (1992). Recognition and management of depression in general practice: Consensus statement. *British Medical Journal*, 305, 1198–1202.

Paykel, E.S., Ramana, R., Cooper, Z., Hayhurst, H., Kerr, J., & Barocka, A. (1995). Residual symptoms after partial remission: An important outcome in depression. *Psychological Medicine*, 25, 1171–1180.

Paykel, E.S., Scott, J., Teasdale, J.D., Johnson, A.L., Garland, A., Moore, R., et al. (1999). Prevention of relapse in residual depression by cognitive therapy: A controlled trial. *Archives of General Psychiatry*, 56, 829–835.

Pearlstein, T., Stone, A., Lund, S., Scheft, H., Zlotnik, C., & Brown, W. (1997). Comparison of fluoxetine, bupropion, and placebo in the treatment of premenstrual dysphoric disorder. *Journal of Clinical Psychopharmacology*, 17, 261–266.

Post, R.M. (1992). Transduction of psychosocial stress into the neurobiology of recurrent affective disorder. *American Journal of Psychiatry*, 149, 999–1010.

Rado, S. (1951). Psychodynamics of depression from the etiologic point of view. *Psychosomatic Medicine,* 13, 51–55.

Rafanelli, C., Park, S.K., & Fava, G.A. (1999). New psychotherapeutic approaches to residual symptoms and relapse prevention in unipolar depression. *Clinical Psychology and Psychotherapy*, 6, 194–201.

Rehm, L.P., & Tyndall, C.I. (1993). Mood disorders: Unipolar and bipolar. In P.B. Sutker & H.E. Adams (Eds.), *Handbook of Psychopathology* (pp. 235–262). New York: Plenum.

Roberts, J.E., Gotlib, I.H., & Kassel, J.D. (1996). Adult attachment security and symptoms of depression: The mediating roles of dysfunctional attitudes and low self-esteem. *Journal of Personality & Social Psychology*, 60, 310–320.

Robins, L.N., & Regier, D.A. (Eds.) (1991). *Psychiatric Disorders in America: The Epidemiologic Catchment Area Study*. New York: Free Press.

Rovner, B.W. (1993). Depression and increased risk of mortality in the nursing home patient. *American Journal of Medicine*, 94, 195–225.

Seligman, M.E.P. (1975). *Helplessness: On Depression, Development of Death*. San Francisco: W.H. Freeman.

Sheline, Y.I. (2000). 3D MRI studies of neuroanatomic changes in unipolar depression major depression: The role of stress and medical comorbidity. *Biological Psychiatry*, 48, 793–800.

Smith, A.L., & Weissman, M.M. (1992). Epidemiology. In E.S. Paykel (Ed.), *Handbook of Affective Disorders*, 2nd ed. (pp. 111–129). London: Churchill Livingstone.

Solomon, D.A., Keller, M.B., Leon, A.C., Mueller, T.I., Lavori, P.W., Shea, T., et al. (2000). Multiple recurrences of major depressive disorder. *American Journal of Psychiatry*, 157(2), 229–233.

Stolberg, R.A., Clark, D.C., & Bongar, B. (2002). Epidemiology, assessment, and management of suicide in depressed patients. In I.H. Gotlib & C.L. Hammen (Eds.), *Handbook of Depression* (pp. 581–601). New York: Guilford Press.

Teicher, M.H., Glod, C., & Cole, J.O. (1990). Emergence of intense suicidal preoccupation during fluoxetine treatment. *American Journal of Psychiatry*, 147(1), 207–210.

Veenstra-VanderWeele, J., Anderson, G.M., & Cook, E.H., Jr. (2000). Pharmacogenetics and the serotonin system: Initial studies and future directions. *European Journal of Pharmacology*, 410(2/3), 165–181.

Wade, T.J., & Cairney, J. (2000). Major depressive disorder and marital transition among mothers: Results from a national panel study. *Journal of Nervous and Mental Disease*, 188, 741–750.

Watts, N.F., & Nicoli, A.M. (1979). Early death of a parent as an etiological factor in schizophrenia. *American Journal of Orthopsychiatry*, 49, 465–473.

Weissman, M.M., Klerman, G.L., & Paykel, E.S. (1971). Clinical evaluation of hostility in depression. *American Journal of Psychiatry*, 128, 261–266.

Wildes, J.E., Harkness, K.L., & Simons, A.D. (2002). Life events, number of social relationships, and twelve-month naturalistic course of major depression in a community sample of women. *Depression and Anxiety*, 16, 104–113.

World Health Organization (1998). *Well-being Measures in Primary Healthcare / The Depcare Project*. Copenhagen: WHO Regional Office for Europe.

# Cognitive Theory
# of Depression

## INTRODUCTION

Depression has been traditionally viewed as an affective disorder, and disordered mood is considered the cardinal symptom, responsible for the patient's behavioral, cognitive, and psychological deficits. The last chapter described how most research has concentrated on finding *either* a biological or psychological cause of depression. Because this research approach is not integrative, it fails to recognize the subtle psychological processes that may cause and maintain the disorder. To break away from this tradition, Aaron Beck has concentrated on the behavioral aspects of depression and has attempted to move beyond description to explain the development and maintenance of depression. Specifically, Beck has emphasized the role of distorted information processing in the pathogenesis of depression. His goal was to develop a theory of depression that fits the patient's behavior, rather than making the patient's behavior fit his theory. He focused on the depressed person's internal world, to understand how he perceives and organizes information and how these formulations affect his symptoms. While positing his cognitive theory of depression, Beck developed a revolutionary new approach (cognitive therapy) to the treatment of depression. Although many cognitive theories of depression exist, this book focuses on Beck's theory because it has generated substantial empirical research on the psychopathology and psychological treatment of depression. This chapter provides a detailed description of Beck's theory of depression, then critically examines the strengths and limitations of cognitive therapy.

## Beck's Cognitive Theory of Depression

According to Beck (1967), the most salient psychological symptom of depression is the profoundly altered thinking or *cognition*. From his extensive clinical experience with treatment of depressive conditions, drawing specifically from his observations of the content and form of depressed patients' dreams and verbalizations, Beck noted that clinically depressed individuals characteristically engage in a negative evaluation of themselves, their environment, and the future. They tend to be constantly preoccupied with these negative thoughts in an almost stereotypic fashion, irrespective of contrary evidence. Such negative thinking is not simply random, but forms a habitual pattern of reference to irrational assumptions or faulty cause–effect relationship that invariably involves inadequate reality testing. These observations led Beck to postulate the hypothesis that the depressed person's cognition is primary in the etiology and manifestation of the symptoms of depression. His theory does not state that faulty or negative cognitions are the *causes* of depression; it simply asserts that such cognitive activity is a primary determinant of the affective and behavioral components of depression.

During the past 30 years, Beck's theory has become more complex and less purist; that is, other cognitive theories of depression (e.g., hopelessness theory of depression) have evolved and, consequently, some aspects of these theories have been integrated with Beck's theory. Moreover, new developments have occurred in general theories of psychopathology. For example, the diathesis-stress or biopsychosocial model of mental illness has become more widely acceptable, and this has been embraced by Beck. Within the context of these developments, Beck's current theory of depression is based on four assumptions (Kuyken, Watkins, & Beck, 2005):

- Depression is a biopsychosocial disorder.
- Maladaptive beliefs originate from childhood experiences.
- Maladaptive beliefs are dormant or unconscious, activated by stressors.
- Maladaptive beliefs interact with precipitating factors to produce depressive symptoms.

The rest of this chapter discusses the basic components of Beck's theory of depression and examines the validity of these assumptions. Because more than 20 therapies are called "cognitive" or "cognitive-behavioral," an explanation to specify what is meant by cognitive therapy is in order. In this book, *cognitive behavior therapy (CBT)* refers to the theory, therapy, and conceptual models developed by Beck and his associates (Beck, 1976; Beck, Rush, et al., 1979). Although the therapy is called "cognitive," its emphasis is on the interaction among five elements: biology, affect, behavior, cognition, and the environment (including developmental history and culture). Because Beck paid close attention to the impact of thinking on affect, behavior, biology, and the experience of the environment, the therapy is called "cognitive." Unfortunately, CBT carries several misunderstandings:

*Cognition causes affect and/or behavior.* Many therapists and writers believe the cognitive models of psychological disorders attribute causation to thinking. This is a myth. CBT considers thoughts, feelings, behaviors, biology, and the environment to be interactive and capable of influencing each other. Thoughts are emphasized because Beck's research demonstrated that dysfunctional thinking can often serve to maintain negative affect. Moreover, extensive empirical evidence suggests that changes in thinking can lead to changes in affect and/or behavior. For these reasons, thoughts are seen as a key target for intervention.

*CBT is purely cognitive.* Although CBT emphasizes the importance of cognition in therapy, close attention is also paid to affect and behavior. Beck, et al. (1979) has highlighted the importance of feelings in cognitive therapy and, more recently, Beck (1991) stated that CBT cannot be conducted in the absence of affect.

***CBT is superficial.*** Some critics have charged that CBT is superficial because it focuses on symptomatic changes. This is not accurate. Although CBT emphasizes here-and-now problems, and teaches patients methods for resolving current problems and sources of distress, the therapy operates at three levels: automatic thoughts, underlying assumptions, and schemas. *Automatic or surface thoughts* are ideas, beliefs, and images related to specific situations that people have each moment (e.g., "My husband did not call, he doesn't really care"). *Underlying assumptions* are deeper levels of thinking, consisting of conditional rules and cross-situational beliefs (e.g., "You can't rely on men"). Our perceptions are organized by these rules, and they form the basis for automatic thoughts. Finally, *schemas* are core beliefs, and they consist of inflexible unconditional beliefs (e.g., "No one really cares for me"). The main goal in CBT is to identify and restructure deeper core beliefs.

***CBT is bullying.*** Because patients are encouraged to confront their dysfunctional thinking, the therapist is never disrespectful of the patient. On the contrary, CBT is considered to be "collaborative empiricism" (Beck, et al., 1979). CBT seeks to form a partnership between the therapist and the patient as they work together collaboratively to understand and solve the patient's problems. Data are collected in an empirical manner to evaluate the evidence for and against dysfunctional and functional beliefs.

### Tripartite Theory of Depressive Cognition

Beck has identified three major clinical features of cognition in depression: (1) the cognitive triad, (2) negative premises and self-schemas, and (3) faulty information processing. The essential components of these cognitive features are briefly described here (for a fuller exposition of these concepts see Beck, et al., 1979).

### *The Cognitive Triad*

The cognitive triad consists of three major dysfunctional cognitive patterns that induce depressed patients to regard themselves, their experiences, and their future in a very negative manner. Beck (1987) considers the cognitive triad to be an intrinsic part of the depressive experience, and at least one aspect of the triad appears to be elevated during a depressive episode.

The first pattern of the cognitive triad revolves around the patient's *negative view of himself*. He regards himself as a failure and as being defective, deprived, inadequate, undesirable, and worthless. He believes that his depression and suffering are caused by some underlying defects within himself and, because of these personal defects, he will never be able to lead a "normal" and happy life, and will always be rejected and disliked by others. Hence he perceives himself as worthless and incapable of achieving happiness.

The second component of the cognitive triad relates to *negative view of the world*. This consists of the tendency of the depressed patient to view the world as hostile, demanding, and obstructive, and thus making it difficult for him to reach his goals in life. Any upset or frustration caused by the interaction with the animate or inanimate environment is seen as defeat or deprivation.

According to Haaga, Dyck, and Ernst (1991), the negative view of the world does not represent the actual state of the world, but one's personal idiosyncratic view of the world.

The third component of the cognitive triad consists of a *negative view of the future*. Depressed patients believe their current suffering, hardship, failure, and deprivation will continue endlessly. Therefore, they anticipate failure in any immediate or future task, leading to a sense of passivity, inertia, and sense of hopelessness.

Other cardinal signs and symptoms of the depressive syndrome are regarded as consequences of the activation of this negative cognitive triad. For example, if a patient erroneously believes that he is a social outcast, then he will feel sad and withdrawn; he will incorrectly believe that he will be disliked or hated and unaccepted by others. This eventually leads to actual feelings of rejection—sadness and loneliness—which are the affective components of depression. The motivational symptoms, such as paralysis of the will, escape and avoidance, wishes, and the like are seen to result from the person's sense of pessimism and hopelessness. In this example, since the person expects a negative outcome (rejection), he will refrain from initiating social contacts, thus increasing his sense of pessimism and hopelessness. Occasionally, the will may become so crippled that the patient contemplates suicide. According to Beck, et al. (1979), suicidal wishes represent an extreme expression of the desire to escape from what appears to be an insoluble problem or an unbearable situation. These feelings result in the depressed person seeing himself as worthless and a burden; consequently he believes that everyone, including himself, will be better off if he is dead.

Increased dependency can also be explained as a consequence of negative cognitions. Because depressed persons regard themselves as incompetent and useless, and because they view the world as presenting insurmountable difficulties, they anticipate failure even in normal tasks. Thus, they feel helpless and need to seek help and reassurance from others, whom they consider more competent and capable than themselves.

Physical symptoms can also be explained as consequences of the negative cognitive process. If patients firmly believe that they are doomed to fail in all efforts, then they are likely to become apathetic. This sense of futility in the future can lead to low energy and inhibition, ultimately resulting in psychomotor retardation.

The negative view of the self and the negative view of the future have been found to be associated with suicide risk (Weishaar & Beck, 1992). Beck found hopelessness or the extreme negative view of the future to be the key psychological factors in suicidality. *Hopelessness* can be defined as a stable schema incorporating negative expectancies. Beck and his colleagues (Beck, Weissman, Lester, & Trexler, 1974; Beck, Steer, Kovacs, & Garrison, 1985; Beck, Brown, Berchick, Stewart, & Steer, 1990) developed the Beck Hopelessness Scale and, through longitudinal research, substantiated the association between hopelessness and suicide risk. They demonstrated the relationship between high levels of hopelessness and suicidal intent. Beck's research in the field of suicide is considered to be one of his most important theoretical and clinical contributions. His conceptualization of suicidality in terms of hopelessness and cognitive distortions provides practical strategies for dealing with suicidal patients.

### Negative Premises and Negative Self-Schemas

The second major ingredient of Beck's theory consists of the concepts of *premises* and *self-schemas*, which he uses to integrate his theory and to explain why some people develop clinical depression and others do not, given the same internal and external event. These concepts also help explain why a depressed patient continues to maintain her pain-inducing and self-defeating attitudes despite objective evidence or positive encounters in her life. These concepts, by virtue of being hypothetical constructs, introduce a certain weakness to Beck's theory, although they can be operationalized and indirectly tested.

*Premises* are implicit or explicit statement of fact that form the basis or cornerstone of an argument, conclusion, evaluation, or problem-solving strategy. From his extensive observation of depressed patients' verbalizations, such as persistent and indiscriminate use of "should" or "must" statements (e.g., "I should be punished"; "I must never fail"), stereotypic conclusions ("It's my fault"), and repeated themes ("I can never succeed"; "I'll never be right") irrespective of the nature of the stimuli, Beck has extrapolated that depressogenic premises or assumptions underlie the patients' negative evaluations.

Negative *self-schemas* or dysfunctional *core beliefs* are learned through such negative childhood experiences as rejection, neglect, abandonment, or abuse. Neisser (1967) defines a *schema* as a relatively enduring structure that functions like a template to active screen, code, categorize, and evaluate incoming information and prior experiences. It consists of bits of information, conclusions, and silent assumptions or premises. Existent self-schemas are highly personalized, and they determine how an individual will structure different experiences. Depressogenic schemas often contain themes of rejection, abandonment, deprivation, defeat, loss, or worthlessness.

Dysfunctional schemas are latent during stable or less stressful times, but can be reactivated by negative experiences that resemble the conditions under which the original beliefs evolved. The response of a person is, therefore, not determined by the event per se, but by the activation of the underlying self-schema. Beck postulates that the activation of latent negative self-schemas are responsible for the depressive states. In his model, a schema serves the dual function of acting as a template or sensor for the selective entry or alteration of incoming stimulation, and for maintaining the internal integrity and consistency of cognitive experience over time by censoring input incongruent to the template.

In depression, the patient's conceptualization of specific situations is distorted to fit the prepotent dysfunctional (negative) schemas. In other words, the active operation of these idiosyncratic schemas interferes with the congruent matching of an appropriate schema to a particular stimulus. Beck, et al. (1979) maintain that, as these idiosyncratic schemas progressively become more active, they gradually generalize to a wider and often unrelated set of stimuli. Consequently, the patient loses much of his voluntary control over his thinking processes and is unable to invoke other more appropriate schemas (this cognitive process is described as a form of negative self-hypnosis in Chapter 4). The repetitive and chronic nature of depressive cognitions and associated symptomatology is attributed to the pervasive influence of negative self-schemas. The depressive syndrome, including the motivational, behavioral, motor, and vegetative symptoms, is believed to be triggered by the activation of this constellation of negative cognitions. The noncognitive components of the depressive syndrome are thus considered secondary to and, to some extent, maintained by the activation of negative cognitive schemas.

## Faulty Information Processing

Faulty information processing or cognitive errors are distorted interpretations of events or situations used by depressed persons to maintain their belief in the validity of their negative self-schemas, despite the presence of contradictory evidence. Beck (1967) has delineated a number of systematic errors of thinking, which depressed patients use to maintain their stereotypic negative conclusions. Burns (1999) has adapted the earlier work by Beck, extending Beck's original postulates to ten systematic errors of thinking or cognitive distortions commonly made by depressed individuals (see Table 2.1). These cognitive distortions are autonomous, plausible, and idiosyncratic; hence, they are referred to as "automatic thoughts" (the concept of negative self-hypnosis discussed in Chapter 4 is very akin to this process).

## Empiric Evidence for Beck's Theory of Depression

Beck's cognitive theory has generated several testable hypotheses about clinical depression. The empirical evidence for some of the key hypotheses is summarized in this section (for reviews, see Hass & Fitzgibbon, 1989; Haaga, Dyck, & Ernst, 1991; and Solomon & Haaga, 2004).

## Depressed Patients Have a Negative Self-Schema

Beck's (1967) cognitive theory assumes that a depressed patient's perception, registration, organization, and recall of incoming information are influenced by negative self-schemas. According to this theory, it is hypothesized that depressed persons would show a bias toward the perception and recall of negative-valence information regarding the self. Haaga, Dyck, and Ernst (1991), from their review of the hypothesis that depressed patients have more negative thoughts than do nondepressed people, conclude that depressed patients have more negative cognitions than nondepressed people. These findings support the hypothesis that negative self-schemas influence information-processing among depressed patients.

## Depressed Patients Have Negative Self-Esteem

Beck proposes that depression is, in part, maintained by negative self-esteem and negative self-image. Self-esteem or sense of personal worth is considered to be a conscious cognitive evaluation of the *self* congruous with the self-schemas. The self is viewed as an organized memory structure containing representational self-referent material (Kuiper & Olinger, 1986). Several studies of self-esteem and depression have shown depressed patients to score

**Table 2.1.  Systematic errors of thinking in depression
(adapted from Burns, 1999)**

**All-or-nothing thinking**
Things are seen as black or white; there is no gray or middle
ground. Things are good or bad, wonderful or awful and, if
performance falls short of perfect, it is a total failure. For example,
if a meal does not turn out to be perfect, the depressed housewife
may conclude: "I can't even cook, I'm no good, I'm a total failure."

**Overgeneralization**
A single negative event is seen as a never-ending pattern of defeat.
If there is a misunderstanding or a disagreement with a person who
is regarded as important (for example, a husband), it is assumed by
the wife that he does not understand or care about her, never has,
and never will. Therefore the wife thinks she will always be
isolated and misunderstood: "No one understands or cares about
me."

**Mental filter or selective abstraction**
A single negative detail is picked out from an event or situation,
and the person dwells on it until everything is darkened, like a drop
of ink that discolors the entire beaker of water. If a housewife
makes a nice dinner, but adds a bit too much dressing on the salad,
then she thinks only of the ruined salad until she sees the entire
dinner party as a disaster: "I ruined everything."

**Disqualifying the positive**
Positive experiences are rejected by insisting they "don't count" for
some reason or another. In this way, a negative belief is maintained,
although it's not based on everyday experiences. For example, a
person may not allow himself to enjoy good feelings because she
believes bad feelings will follow if she allows herself to feel good.
Thus, she even feels bad about feeling good: "I'm afraid to feel
happy because I always feel bad afterward."

**Jumping to conclusions or arbitrary inferences**
Negative interpretations are made, although there are no definite
facts to support the conclusions. A person jumps to conclusions
either by *mind reading* or *fortune telling*.

a. *Mind Reading*: A tendency to see things as negative, but not
bothering to check out the facts. For example, if a coworker does
not say "Good morning," a depressed person may conclude the
coworker dislikes her; she gets upset about it and does not bother
to check whether the coworker himself is upset or worried about
something.

b. *Fortune Teller Error*: Anticipates that things will turn out badly
and does not allow for the possibility that they may be neutral
or positive. In other words, a negative prediction is treated as an
established fact: "No need to take the exam, I'm sure I'll fail" or
"I'll not enjoy the party so what's the point in going?"

(continued)

## Table 2.1.   (Continued)

**Magnification and/or minimization**
This is also called the "binocular trick." An extra big deal is made about personal errors and an extra big deal is made about other people's success. At the same time, it is maintained that other people's errors don't really matter, and that personal successes and good qualities are really small and don't count for much. In other words, the importance of things is exaggerated or inappropriately diminished. "I made a mistake, I'm so stupid"; "They say I have a good home, this doesn't count, anyone can have a home."

**Emotional reasoning**
It is assumed that negative feelings result from the fact that things *are* negative. If a person feels bad, then it means the situation is bad. The depressed person does not bother to check if things are really bad. "I feel rejected, therefore, it must be true that people don't like me."

**Should statements**
This refers to the tendency of trying to push or improve oneself with *shoulds* and *shouldn'ts*, *musts* and *oughts*. For example, "I should do more"; "I should have known better"; "I must not fail"; "I ought to be a good father"; "I should have done the right thing." The emotional consequences of these statements are guilt, anger, and resentment. *Should* statements are often used when "I wish" or "I would like to" or "It would have been desirable" would have been more appropriate.

**Labeling and mislabeling**
This is an extreme form of overgeneralization. Instead of describing an error or mistake, a negative label is attached to the self: "I said the wrong thing, I'm so dumb." When someone disagrees or disproves one's point of view, the person is negatively labeled: "He's horrible, he's repulsive," rather than "he disagrees with my opinion." Labeling and mislabeling involves describing an event or person in emotionally loaded language. Such description severely restricts the focus of attention to a few isolated details and makes inferences to characteristics unrelated to a particular person or situation.

**Personalization**
One sees oneself as the cause of some external unfortunate or unpleasant event for which, in fact, one is not actually responsible. A woman, for example, who was emotionally and physically abused as a child blames herself for these "bad things" because she believes she is a bad person and "was born bad."

---

lower on measures of self-esteem (e.g., Feather, 1983) and higher on measures of self-consciousness (Sacco & Hokanson, 1978) than nondepressed people.

### Depressed Patients Have a Greater Sense of Self-Blame
Consistent with their negative self-schemas, depressed patients tend to have negative self-images, supported by feelings of inadequacy, ineffectuality, and self-blame (Beck, 1967). This

position is, however, regarded as a theoretical paradox. On one hand, depressed patients are viewed as blaming themselves for any negative outcome; on the other hand, they are described as perceiving little control over personal outcomes (Peterson, 1979). Abramson and Sackheim (1977) have attributed this apparent contradiction to the depressed person's tendency to isolate or split off his feelings of omnipotence from his feelings of impotence. Peterson (1979), from his study of the association between self-blame and attributions of internal versus external locus of control, has concluded that depressed patients tend to show a type of illogical thinking characterized by attributions of external control (i.e., stable tendency to infer external source of control over personal events) while indulging in habitual self-blame. Other writers such as Haas and Fitzgibbon (1989) have suggested that self-blame may be more adequately understood as a form of self-punitive behavior maintained independently of the cognitive perception of the uncontrollability of specific personal events.

### Depressed Patients Have a Negative Self-Perception of Coping Adequacy

Self-blaming may also represent a tendency among depressed persons to blame the self for failure to exert control under circumstances of stress. In several studies, it has been consistently found that depressed patients are more self-critical, endorse more negative and fewer positive self-descriptive adjectives, report lower self-esteem, and rate themselves as more discrepant from their ideal selves (see review by Haaga, et al., 1991). Moreover, depressed patients express higher levels of hopelessness related to coping adequacy (Rush, Beck, Kovacs, Weinberger, & Hollon, 1982).

### Depressed Patients Have a Negative View of the Future

A negative view of the future forms part of the cognitive triad. According to Beck, depressed patients have the tendency to view current unpleasant conditions as continuing and future or new events to have negative outcomes. Several studies have demonstrated that depressed patients are more hopeless about the future than are nondepressed or remitted depressed people (e.g., Dohr, et al., 1989). Other studies have revealed a correlation between negative cognition about future outcomes and depression (e.g., Fibel & Hale, 1978; Raps, Peterson, Reinhard, Abramson & Seligman, 1982). Although the temporal relationship between pessimistic outlook and depression cannot be inferred from the data, these studies consistently show pessimistic attitude to be a characteristic of clinically depressed states.

### Depressed Patients Have a Negative View of the World

Another aspect of the cognitive triad relates to a person's view of the world. Beck (1967, 1976) contends that depressed people have a negative view of the external world. Greenberg and Beck (1989) examined the world component of the cognitive triad with a sample of depressed and nondepressed psychiatric patients and found depressed patients to endorse more depressive adjectives regarding the world than did the psychiatric control group.

### Cognitive Triad Is Universal to All Subtypes of Depression

Beck (1991) has posited a *universality hypothesis*, the contention that all subtypes of clinical depression have similar negative cognitions. Several studies have corroborated Beck's observation that depressive cognitions are similar across the traditional nosologic categories of depressions (see review by Haaga, et al., 1991).

### Depressed Patients Have Specific Cognitive Distortions

Beck has proposed the *content-specificity* hypothesis, which maintains that, although negativity is common to all emotional disorders, each disorder has its own specific set of cognitive distortion. Several investigators found depressed patients to score higher on the Automatic Thought Questionnaire than heterogeneous nondepressed psychiatric patients (e.g., Dobson & Shaw, 1986). Because of the frequent comorbidity of depression with anxiety (Dozois & Westra, 2004), many investigators have compared the cognitive contents of anxious and depressed patients. The findings indicate that depressed patients are more preoccupied with loss, defeat, and negative outcomes, whereas anxious patients are more concerned with threat and danger (Beck, et al., 1987; Greenberg & Beck, 1989). Moreover, a factor analytic study of all the cognitive scales designed to assess cognitive content of depression and anxiety yielded appropriate loadings on anxiety and depression factors (Clark, Beck, & Brown, 1989).

### Depressed Patients Show Biases in Perception and Recall

Apart from the extensive literature on the association between faulty information-processing (cognitive distortions) and depression, various studies have supported Beck's assumption that depressed patients show cognitive distortions or biases (e.g., Carver & Ganellen, 1983; Hamilton & Abramson, 1983) that are in excess of nondepressed controls (Blaney, et al., 1980).

### Depressed Patients Have Automatic Negative Cognitions

According to Beck, negative cognitions are automatic, repetitive, and not readily controllable. Moretti and Shaw (1989) argue that the processes leading to automatic thoughts may be automatic, but the thoughts themselves occupy considerable attention. No research has tested automaticity and unintentionality in clinical depression. Research with subclinical dysphoric subjects, however, does show automatic information processing about the self (Bargh & Tota, 1988).

### The Degree of Depressive Cognitive and Noncognitive Symptoms Are Related

The cognitive theory of depression asserts that the degree of negative cognitions is associated with the severity of noncognitive symptoms of depression. Many studies found high correlation between depressive cognition measures and self-reported depressive symptoms (e.g., Dent & Teasdale, 1988). Similarly several cross-sectional studies demonstrated that hopelessness is positively correlated with suicidal intent (e.g., Beck, Brown, & Steer, 1989). From the existing evidence, it appears severity of negative cognitions is correlated positively with the severity of noncognitive symptoms (Haaga, et al., 1991).

## Cognitive Restructuring Leads to Reduction in Depressive Symptoms

Based on his theory, Beck devised CBT to help depressed patients replace maladaptive cognitive processes with more adaptive cognitions. Since the treatment procedures are well-operationalized, they are amenable to controlled study. CBT is the most extensively tested psychosocial treatment for depression. It has been studied in over 80 controlled trials (American Psychiatric Association, 2000), and it has been found to be effective in reducing acute distress. It compares favorably with pharmacologic treatment among all but the most severely depressed patients. Moreover, CBT reduces relapse and can prevent the initial onset of first episodes or the emergence of symptoms in persons at risk who have never been depressed (Gillham, Shatte, & Freres, 2000). Although it is unclear precisely how CBT produces positive effect, Hollon, et al. (2002) believe symptomatic relief is due to changes in core beliefs and information-processing proclivities. Goldapple, et al. (2004) have provided functional neuroimaging (positron emission tomography, or PET) evidence to demonstrate that CBT produces specific cortical regional changes in treatment responders. While CBT produced significant directional changes in the frontal cortex, cingulate, and hippocampus, an SSRI antidepressant medication (specifically paroxetine) produced significant changes in the limbic and subcortical regions (brainstem, insula, and subgenual cingulate). The authors concluded that CBT "like other antidepressant treatments affect clinical recovery by modulating the functioning of specific sites in limbic and cortical regions" (p. 34).

### Conclusions from Empirical Studies of Beck's Theory

In conclusion, empirical studies support the presence of several cognitive changes associated with clinical depression. However, they do not provide unequivocal evidence of cognitive factors in the etiology and pathogenesis of depression.

### Predisposition and Maintenance of Depression

The cognitive theory of depression also offers a hypothesis about the predisposition and maintenance of clinical depression. Beck asserts that childhood experiences provide the basis for forming deep-seated negative schemas about some aspect of life (Young, Weinberger, & Beck, 2001). With a "self-blame" schema, individuals feel personally responsible for every bad thing that happens (personalization). With a negative "self-evaluation" schema, individuals believe they can never do anything correctly (overgeneralization, disqualifying the positives). These self-schemas may be latent or unconscious, but can be automatically activated by specific circumstances analogous to the original experiences that shaped the initial negative cognitions. For example, depression can be triggered by separation from a spouse. Here the separation activated the person's latent concept of irreversible loss associated with the death of a parent during childhood. However, events that activate dysphoric feelings do not, in and of themselves, cause depression. The events simply act as "triggers" for the onset of clinical depression in persons with a cognitive predisposition (i.e., persons with negative self-schemas).

Several empirical studies support the hypothesis that individuals with latent negative schemas are vulnerable for depression (e.g., Gotlib & Krasnoperova, 1998). There is also a significant body of data supporting Beck's prediction that many depressed individuals have experienced negative events in childhood (see review by Ingram, Miranda, & Segal, 1998). However, it is not easy to test the hypothesis that latent depressive beliefs are diatheses to depression. Since latent depressive beliefs are unavailable to awareness before the onset of depression, they are difficult to measure and verify as predating depression.

As noted before, Beck's theory of depression also attributes the characteristic persistence of negative cognitions and self-defeating behaviors as emanating from the activation of negative self-schemas. Once a negative schema is activated, it influences the interpretation of incoming stimuli to maintain the consistency of the underlying negative cognitive structure. In other words, biased information processing helps to maintain the consistency between experience and self-schemas, thus perpetuating the depressive symptoms. Hence, Beck's depressive model is regarded as a circular model, which is further discussed in Chapter 4.

According to Beck's theory, maladaptive self-schemas containing dysfunctional attitudes involving themes of loss, inadequacy, failure, and worthlessness constitute the cognitive vulnerability for depression. When these depressogenic self-schemas are activated by the occurrence of stressors (negative life-events), they generate specific negative cognitions (automatic thoughts) that galvanize the cognitive triad. This, in turn, leads to dysphoria and depressive symptoms. In the absence of insignificant stressors, the depressogenic self-schemas are unconscious, and they do not trigger negative automatic thoughts or depressive symptoms. Five central predictions emanates from Beck's theory of depression:

- Cognitive vulnerability interacts with stressors to produce symptoms. Individuals who are cognitively vulnerable are more at risk of developing depression than are individuals who do not exhibit cognitive vulnerability when faced with a negative life-event.
- The relationship between depressive symptoms and stressors is mediated by the cognitive triad.
- A chain of events lead to depression.
- The congruency of cognitive vulnerability and negative events increases the likelihood of a depressive episode.
- Depressive cognitions are distorted.

The etiologic hypotheses of the cognitive theories of depression have been empirically investigated. Both retrospective and prospective studies have demonstrated that the cognitive vulnerability × stress interaction (more specifically, dysfunctional attitudes × negative events) predict increases in depressive symptoms over time. The ongoing Cognitive Vulnerability to Depression (CVD) Project, a collaborative two-site study, has been the most comprehensive investigation to test the cognitive vulnerability hypothesis. In this study, undepressed university freshmen at either high or low cognitive risk for depression (measured by Cognitive Style Questionnaire and the Dysfunctional Attitude Scale) were followed for 5 years with self-report and structured interview assessments every 6 weeks to determine if they experienced any stressful life events or diagnosable episodes of depression. The initial findings of the CVD Project provide direct and compelling support for the cognitive vulnerability hypothesis (Alloy, Abramson, Hogan, Whitehouse, Rose, Robinson, et al., 2000). Students at high risk (with dysfunctional attitudes) reported higher rates of depression in the past compared with the low-risk group. The most important results came from the prospective portion of study. Results from the first 2.5 years of follow-up suggest that negative cognitive styles serve as an indicator of later depression. Even if participants had never suffered from depression before in their lives, high-risk participants (who scored high on the measures of cognitive vulnerability) were far more likely than low-risk participants to experience a major depressive episode or at least depressive symptoms. Seventeen percent of the high-risk subjects versus only 1% of the low-risk subjects experienced major depressive episodes, and 39% versus 6% experienced minor depressive symptoms. These data are very suggestive that cognitive vulnerabilities to developing depression do exist and, when combined with biological vulnerabilities, create a slippery path to depression (Barlow & Durand, 2005). However, future research should specify more precisely how cognitive vulnerabilities and stress combine to produce depression.

### Relationship between Cognitive Vulnerability and Rumination

Several investigators (e.g., Nolen-Hoeksema, 1991) have demonstrated that rumination also plays an important role in many aspects of depression. Nolen-Hoeksema posits that rumination represents a process of perseverative attention directed to specific, mainly internal, content. For example, a depressed person may become focused on her negative affect, the causes of the negative feeling, and the consequences of the depressed mood. The tendency to ruminate is associated with several factors including vulnerability to depressed mood, onsets of depressive episodes, longer and more severe depressive episodes, gender differences in depressive vulnerability, and various symptoms of depression (see Abramson, Alloy, Hankin, Haeffel, MacCoon, & Gibb, 2002).

The relationship between cognitive vulnerability and Beck's theory of depression has not been established. Abramson, et al. (2002) have examined the role of rumination in the context of their cognitive vulnerability–stress model of depression. Within this context, they believe cognitive vulnerability leads to rumination. They argue that cognitively vulnerable individuals are at high risk of engaging in rumination. They provide four lines of evidence to support their contention that rumination is a particular type of self-regulatory problem: (i) attention serves as a "spotlight" that selects the "subject" that will influence behavior and mood at a given moment; (ii) when confronted with a negative event, people switch their attention to the problem; (iii) cognitively vulnerable individuals have difficulty disengaging their attention from negative cognitive content; and (iv) rumination with negative cognitive content increases negative affect. The implication of negative rumination in depression is further discussed in the context of negative-self hypnosis in Chapter 4.

## STRENGTHS AND WEAKNESSES OF THE COGNITIVE THEORY AND THERAPY OF DEPRESSION

CBT has many strengths as well as some weaknesses. The strengths and weaknesses of CBT are highlighted to illustrate that none of the theories of depression is able to fully address all the components involved in depression. However, the integrative approach of CBT is superior to treatment using a single model.

### Strengths of CBT

1. Treatment is time-limited. The course of cognitive therapy is generally 12 to 20 sessions. A subtle reminder of time limitation provides an impetus to working concretely on problems of major importance.
2. Cognitive therapy is active, collaborative, interactive, and skills-based. Therapeutic change is attributed to the patient's efforts and usage of specific change strategies, rather than merely to the skills of the therapist.
3. Problems are clearly defined within the cognitive framework, providing a common language to both patient and therapist.
4. Individual sessions, as well as the entire therapeutic process, have a high degree of structure. The course of therapy is structured to initially emphasize assessment, then moves on to a focus on behavior, and finally to cognition—both automatic thoughts and underlying assumptions.
5. Goals are clearly defined, and various targets provided to achieve goals.
6. CBT offers a direct method of modifying feelings (affect), physiological responses, and behaviors. The ability to modify these responses provides patients with confidence and sense of self-control.
7. Treatment is concerned with the present and here-and-now, and what the patient can actively do to reduce problems and symptoms.
8. Because language or syntax is used for communication, the modification of syntax seems natural.
9. Patients are easily persuaded into changing their thinking. By changing thinking, patients experience instant modification of symptoms, which reinforces the credibility of the cognitive model and results in greater compliance.
10. CBT reduces suicidal ideation, especially in the initial stages of therapy.
11. CBT involves behavioral activities, reading, monitoring and changing maladaptive thoughts, and graded realistic targets. All these tasks aid patients in continual restructuring of their depressogenic schemas outside therapy sessions.
12. The positive effects of CBT are long lasting, and the skills acquired can be extended to coping with other problems, thus preventing future relapses.

13. CBT is equally or more effective than drug therapy. It provides an effective alternative to medication, without the risk of side effects.
14. CBT produces specific cortical changes; therefore, its effect is not superficial.

### Shortcomings of Cognitive Therapy

1. Cognitive therapy is time-consuming. Each session takes approximately an hour, and 12 to 20 sessions are required.
2. It is not effective in very severe depression. Severity should be reduced by other means (drugs or ECT) before instituting CBT.
3. High motivation and maximum commitment is required on the part of both therapist and patient.
4. Some patients, because of their cultural or educational background, are unable to comprehend the cognitive concepts.
5. Despite its demonstrated efficacy, it is still not known how CBT effects change. Understanding this process is a fundamental theoretical challenge and one of great and active interest.
6. Because CBT mainly involves syntax or verbal communication, cognitive therapy is a left-hemispheric process for the majority of people (right handers). Therefore, it has only an indirect influence (less powerful) on the right hemisphere, which may be related to the experience of depression. This implies that CBT may not be very effective when patients are dissociated (right hemisphere engagement); that is, they will not be attending to the therapist while covertly involved in their imagination.
7. CBT makes little use of the imaginal processes (since the emphasis is on syntax). Imaginal processes are increasingly viewed as a constructive activity influencing learning (Pavio, 1971), memory (Bower, 1981; Pavio, 1971), and perception (Segal, 1971). Miller (1984) has reviewed the evidence for the neurophysiological changes brought on by imagery in depression. The work of Schwartz (1976, 1977, 1984) indicates a "normal" person may develop depression by establishing certain neurologic pathways owing to conscious negative mental focus (imagery). These brain patterns, with repeated cognitive focus (imagery), may become consistent, automatic, and unresponsive to cognitive therapy or pharmacotherapy (Miller, 1984). Imagery training (positive cognitive focus) may be more appropriate here. Schultz (1978, 1984) has provided evidence for the short-term benefits of directed imagery in depression, and Singer and Pope (1978) have emphasized the clinical implications of imagery and discussed numerous techniques that have been utilized to augment the treatment of various psychiatric syndromes.
8. CBT ignores the role of unconscious processes. Unconscious processes may be nonverbal and a function of the right hemisphere (Galin, 1974), therefore not directly influenced by syntax.
9. CBT assumes the primacy of cognition; that is, cognition always precedes emotion/affect. Barnett (1979) and Jaynes (1976) have stressed the independence of affect and cognition.

Miller (1984), influenced by these writers, has emphasized the concept of the "bicameral brain" (two-sided brain) in the understanding and treatment of emotional disorders. Bicameral cognition involves conscious accessing of either affect or cognition. Such understanding implies that when a person is consciously accessing affect, her behavior is arising from the cognitive affect, rather than being determined by verbalization (e.g., beliefs of self-talk). In such a situation, verbal restructuring will have little effect on feelings.

10. Although faulty cognition is apparent during depression there is no evidence for the causality of distorted cognition in depression. However, the question remains why or how CBT produces clinical improvement. Coyne (1980) has taken up this issue and offers some alternative ways of conceptualizing the role of cognition in depression. He offers the view that cognition is better conceptualized as a set of relationships that reach out into a larger context of interrelated, loosely fused psychological and physiological processes. Cognitive therapy can be regarded as a technique that provides one of several points of entry into this interrelated system. By "freezing" the cognitive activity, a description of the internal world of the depressed patient is developed. Through cognitive therapy, both patient and therapist can gain access into this set of relationships and, by employing systematic techniques as tools, can unravel and reorganize this set of relationships. Focusing on the cognitive processes as targets for intervention seems to work to influence simultaneously other processes because of their interrelated nature.

   Pharmacotherapy or other forms of therapies may identify points of entry into this system and organize the system using their own processes. A working model of depression providing different entries will be presented in Chapter 4.

11. Cognitive therapy does not explain why nondepressed people with biased perceptions do not develop clinical depression.

12. The cognitive model does not explain the process by which depression remits in the absence of therapy (psychological or pharmacological). In fact, cognitive theory would predict difficulty in overcoming depression if a persistence of negative cognitions exists (Lewinshon, et al., 1981).

13. CBT tends to underplay the beneficial effects of antidepressant drugs in certain forms of depression. Simons, Garfield, and Murphy (1984), in a study comparing the effect of pharmacotherapy with cognitive therapy, demonstrated that medication resulted in cognitive changes comparative to those of cognitive therapy, despite the absence of direct focus on cognitive, behavioral, and physiological processes. Therefore medication, like cognitive therapy, is capable of reorganizing this constellation of processes. However, simply because medication works does not necessarily mean biochemistry comes first and all else follows. It is more likely that the modification of one facet of the whole picture affects the rest of the system.

## SUMMARY

Beck's cognitive theory of depression and his innovative approach to treatment were critically examined in this chapter. Specifically,

Beck's theory is based on four main assumptions (Kuyken, Watkins, & Beck, 2005): (a) depression is a biopsychosocial disorder; (b) maladaptive beliefs originate from childhood experiences; (c) these maladaptive beliefs are dormant or unconscious but can be activated by stressors; and (d) maladaptive beliefs interact with precipitating factors to produce depressive symptoms. Although Beck did not focus on clarifying the etiology of depression, his model provides a window for entering and rearranging the depressive world. However, there is evidence that the effect of CBT is augmented by integrating it with hypnotherapy (Alladin, 2005, 2006; Alladin & Alibhai, 2007). Chapter 4 presents an integrative model of depression and Part III of the book describes a multimodal approach for dealing with depression.

**REFERENCES**

Abramson, L.Y., Alloy, L.B., Hankin, B.L., Haeffel, G.J., MacCoon, D.G., & Gibb, B.E. (2002). Cognitive-vulnerability – Stress models of depression in a self-regulatory and psychobiological context. In I.H. Gotlib & C.L. Hammen (Eds.), *Handbook of depression* (pp. 268–294). New York: Guilford Press.

Abramson, L.Y., & Sackheim, H.A. (1977). A paradox in depression: Uncontrollability and self-blame. *Psychology Bulletin*, 84, 838–851.

Alladin, A. (2005). *Cognitive hypnotherapy for depression: An empirical investigation*. Paper presented at the American Psychological Association Annual Convention, August 2005.

Alladin, A. (2006). Cognitive hypnotherapy for treating depression. In R. Chapman (Ed.), *The clinical use of hypnosis with cognitive behavior therapy: A practitioner's casebook* (pp. 139–187). New York: Springer Publishing Company.

Alladin, A., & Alibhai, A. (2007). Cognitive hypnotherapy therapy for depression: An empirical investigation. *International Journal of Clinical and Experimental Hypnosis*, in press.

Alloy, L.B., Abramson, L.Y., Hogan, M.E., Whitehouse, W.G., Rose, D.T., Robinson, M.S., et al. (2000). The Temple-Wisconsin Cognitive Vulnerability to Depression (CVD) Project: Lifetime history of Axis I psychopathology in individuals at high and low cognitive risk for depression. *Journal of Abnormal Psychology*, 109, 403–418.

American Psychiatric Association (2000). *Diagnostic and Statistical Manual of Mental Disorders,* 4th ed., Text Rev. Washington, DC: American Psychiatric Press.

Bargh, J.A., & Tota, M.E. (1988). Context-dependent automatic processing in depression: Accessibility of negative constructs with regard to self but not others. *Journal of Personality and Social Psychology*, 54, 925–939.

Barlow, D.H., & Durand, V.M. (2005). *Abnormal psychology: An integrative approach* (4th edition). Boston: Thomson Wadworth.

Barnett, J. (1979). Character, cognition and therapeutic process. *American Journal of Psychoanalysis*, 39, 291–301.

Beck, A.T. (1967). *Depression: Clinical, experimental and theoretical aspects*. New York: Hoeber.

Beck, A.T. (1976). *Cognitive therapy and emotional disorders*. New York: International University Press.

Beck, A.T. (1991). Cognitive therapy: A 30-year retrospective. *American Psychologist*, 46, 368–375.

Beck, A.T., Brown, G., Berchick, R.J., Stewart, B.L., & Steer, R.A. (1990). Relationship between hopelessness and ultimate suicide: A replication with psychiatric outpatients. *American Journal of Psychiatry*, 147, 190–195.

Beck, A.T., Brown, G., & Steer, R.A. (1989). Prediction of eventual suicide in psychiatric inpatients by clinical ratings of hopelessness. *Journal of Consulting and Clinical Psychology*, 57, 309–310.

Beck, A.T., Brown, G., Steer, R.A., Eidelson, J.I., & Riskind, J.H. (1987). Differentiating anxiety and depression: A test of the cognitive-content-specificity hypothesis. *Journal of Abnormal Psychology*, 96, 179–183.

Beck, A.T., Rush, A.J., Shaw, B.F., & Emery, G. (1979). *Cognitive therapy of depression*. New York: Guilford Press.

Beck, A.T., Steer, R.A., Kovacs, M., & Garrison, B. (1985). Hopelessness and eventual suicide: A 10-year prospective study of patients hospitalized with suicidal ideation. *American Journal of Psychiatry*, 142, 559–563.

Beck, A.T., Weissman, A., Lester, D., & Trexler, L. (1974). The measurement of pessimism: The hopelessness scale. *Consulting Clinical Psychology*, 42, 861–865.

Beck, A.T., & Young, J.E. (1985). Depression. In D.H. Barlow (Ed.), *Clinical handbook of psychological disorders*. New York: Guilford Press.

Blaney, P.H., Behar, V., & Head, R. (1980). Two measures of depressive cognitions: Their association with depression and with each other. *Journal of Abnormal Psychology*, 89, 678–682.

Bower, G. (1981). Mood and memory. *American Psychologist*, 36, 129–148.

Burns, D.D. (1999). *Feeling good: The new mood therapy*. New York: Avon Books.

Carver, C.S., & Ganellen, R.J. (1983). Depression and components of self-punitiveness: High standards, self-criticism, and overgeneralization. *Journal of Consulting and Clinical Psychology*, 92, 330–337.

Clark, D.A., Beck, A.T., & Brown, G. (1989). Cognitive mediation in general psychiatric outpatients: A test of the content-specificity hypothesis. *Journal of Personality and Social Psychology*, 56, 958–964.

Coyne, J.C. (1980). A critique of cognitions as causal entities with particular reference to depression. *Cognitive Therapy and Research*, 6, 3–13.

Dent, J. & Teasdale, J.D. (1988). Negative cognition and the persistence of depression. *Journal of Abnormal Psychology*, 97, 29–34.

Dobson, K.S., & Shaw, B.F. (1986). Cognitive assessment with major depressive disorders. *Cognitive Therapy and Research*, 10, 13–29.

Dohr, K.B., Rush, A.J., & Bernstein, I.H. (1989). Cognitive biases and depression. *Journal of Abnormal Psychology*, 98, 263–267.

Dozois, D.J.A., & Westra, H.A. (2004). The nature of anxiety and depression: Implications for prevention. In D.J.A. Dozois & K.S. Dobson (Eds.), *The prevention of anxiety and depression: Theory, research, and practice* (pp. 9–41). Washington, DC: American Psychological Association.

Feather, N.T. (1983). Some correlates of attributional style: Depressive self-esteem and Protestant ethic values. *Personality and Social Psychology Bulletin*, 9, 125–135.

Fibel, B., & Hale, W.D. (1978). The generalized expectancy for success scale: A new measure. *Journal of Consulting and Clinical Psychology*, 46, 924–931.

Galin, D. (1974). Implications for psychiatry of left and right cerebral specialization. *Archives of General Psychiatry*, 31, 572–583.

Gillham, J.E., Shatte, A.J., & Freres, D.R. (2000). Preventing depression: A review of cognitive-behavioral and family interventions. *Applied and Preventive Psychology*, 9, 63–88.

Goldapple, K., Segal, Z., Garson, C., Lau, M., Bieling, P, Kennedy, S., & Mayberg, H. (2004). Modulation of cortical-limbic pathways in major depression: Treatment-specific effects of cognitive behavior therapy. *Archives of General Psychiatry*, 61, 34–41.

Gotlib, I.H., & Krasnoperova, E. (1998). Biased information processing as a vulnerability factor for depression. *Behavior Therapy*, 29, 603–617.

Greenberg, M.S., & Beck, A.T. (1989). Depression versus anxiety: A test of the content specificity hypothesis. *Journal of Abnormal Psychology*, 98, 9–13.

Haaga, D.A.F., Dyck, M.J., & Ernst, D. (1991). Empirical status of cognitive theory of depression. *Psychological Bulletin*, 110, 215–236.

Haas, G.L., & Fitzgibbon, M.L. (1989). In J.J. Mann (Ed.), *Models of depressive disorders* (pp. 9–43). Plenum Press, New York.

Hamilton, E.W., & Abramson, L.Y. (1983). Cognitive patterns and major depressive disorder: A longitudinal study in a hospital setting. *Journal of Abnormal Psychology*, 92, 173–184.

Hollon, S.D., Haman, K.L., & Brown, L.L. (2002). Cognitive-behavioral treatment of depression. In I.H. Gotlib & C.C. Hammen (Eds.), *Handbook of depression* (pp. 383–403). New York: Guilford Press.

Hollon, S.D., & Shelton, M. (1991). Contributions of cognitive psychology to assessment and treatment of depression. In P.R. Martin (Ed.), *Handbook of behavior therapy and psychological science: An integrated approach* (Vol. 164, pp. 169–195). New York: Pergamon Press.

Ingram, R.E., Miranda, J., & Segal, Z.V. (1998). *Cognitive vulnerability to depression*. New York: Guilford Press.

Jaynes, J. (1976). *The origin of consciousness in the breakdown of the bicameral mind*. Boston: Houghton Mifflin Co.

Kuiper, N.A., & Olinger, L.J. (1986). Dysfunctional attitudes and a self-worth contingency model of depression. In P.C. Kendall (Eds.), *Advances in cognitive-behavioral research and therapy* (Vol. 5, pp. 115–142). Orlando, FL: Academic Press.

Kuyken, W., Watkins, E., & Beck, A.T. (2005). Cognitive-behavior therapy for mood disorders. In G.O. Gabbard, J.S. Beck, & J. Holmes (Eds.), *Oxford Textbook of Psychotherapy* (pp. 111–124). Oxford University Press.

Lewinshon, P.M., Steinmetz, J.L., Larson, D.W., & Frankin, J. (1981). Depression-related cognitions: Antecedent or consequence? *Journal of Abnormal Psychology*, 90, 213–219.

Miller, H.R. (1984). Depression – a specific cognitive pattern. In W.C. Wester & A.H. Smith (Eds.), *Clinical hypnosis: A multidisci-*

*plinary approach* (pp. 421–457). Philadelphia: J.B. Lippincott Company.

Moretti, M.M., & Shaw, B.F. (1989). Automatic and dysfunctional cognitive processes in depression. In J.S. Uleman & J.A. Bargh (Eds.), *Unintended thought* (pp. 383–421). New York: Guilford Press.

Nolen-Hoeksema, S. (1991). Responses to depression and their effects on the duration of depressive episodes. *Journal of Abnormal Psychology*, 100, 569–582.

Pavio, A. (1971). *Imagery and verbal processes*. New York: Holt, Rinehart, and Winston.

Peterson, C. (1979). Uncontrollability and self-blame in depression: Investigation of the paradox in a college population. *Journal of Abnormal Psychology*, 88, 620–624.

Raps, C.S., Peterson, C., Reinhard, K.E., Abramson, L.Y., & Seligman, M.E.P. (1982). Attributional style among depressed patients. *Journal of Abnormal Psychology*, 91, 102–108.

Rush, A.F., Beck, A.T., Kovacs, M., Weinberger, J.A., & Hollon, S.D. (1982). Comparison of the effects of cognitive therapy and pharmacotherapy on hopelessness and self-concept. *American Journal of Psychiatry*, 139, 862–866.

Sacco, W.P., & Hokanson, J.E. (1978). Expectations of success and anagram performance of depressives in a public and private setting. *Journal of Abnormal Psychology*, 87, 122–130.

Schultz, K.D. (1978). Imagery and the control of depression. In J.L. Singer & K.S. Pope (Eds.), *The power of human imagination: New methods in psychotherapy* (pp. 281–307). New York: Plenum Press.

Schultz, K.D. (1984) The use of imagery in alleviating depression. In A.A. Sheik (Ed.), *Imagination and healing* (pp. 129–158). Amityville NY: Baywood Publishing Co.

Schwartz, G. (1976). Facial muscle patterning in affective imagery in depressed and non-depressed subjects. *Science*, 192, 489–491.

Schwartz, G. (1977). Psychosomatic disorders in biofeedback: A psychological model of disregulation. In J.D. Maser & M.E.P. Seligman (Eds.), *Psychopathology: Experimental models* (pp. 270–307). San Francisco: W.H. Freeman.

Schwartz, G. (1984). Psychophysiology of imagery and healing: A systems perspective. In A.A. Sheik (Ed.), *Imagination and healing* (pp. 35–50). Amityville NY: Baywood Publishing Co.

Segal, S.J. (Ed.) (1971). *Imagery: Current cognitive approaches*. New York: Academic Press.

Simons, A.D., Garfield, S.L., & Murphy, G.E. (1984). The process of change in cognitive therapy and pharmacotherapy for depression. *Archives of General Psychiatry*, 41, 45–51.

Singer, J.L., & Pope, K.S. (1978). The use of imagery and fantasy techniques in psychotherapy. In J.L. Singer & K.S. Pope (Eds.), *The power of human imagination: New methods in psychotherapy* (pp. 3–34). New York: Plenum Press.

Solomon, A., & Haaga, D.A.F. (2004). Cognitive theory and therapy of depression. In M.A. Reinecke & D.A. Clark (Eds.), *Cognitive therapy across the lifespan: Evidence and practice* (pp. 12–39). Cambridge University Press.

Weishaar, M.E., & Beck, A.T. (1992). Clinical and cognitive predictors of suicide. In R.W. Maris, A.L. Berman, J.T. Mattsberger, & R.I.

Yufit (Eds.), *Assessment and prediction of suicide* (pp. 467–483). New York: Guilford Press.

Young, J.E., Weinberger, A.D., & Beck, A.T. (2001). Cognitive therapy for depression, In D.H. Barlow (Ed.), *Clinical handbook of psychological disorders* (3rd ed., pp. 264–308). New York: Guilford Publications.

# Hypnosis and Hypnotherapy

This chapter briefly reviews the neodissociation theory of hypnosis, and the limitations and strengths of clinical hypnosis. Although many contemporary theories of hypnosis exist, the focus here is on the neodissociation theory of hypnosis as it forms part of the cognitive-dissociative model of depression (CDMD) described in Chapter 4.

## THEORIES OF HYPNOSIS

Hypnosis, in one form or another, has been used in different parts of the world to treat various medical and psychological disorders since ancient times. In the 18th century, Franz Anton Mesmer, a physician from Vienna, conceptualized hypnotherapy as a formal form of psychotherapy for a variety of psychological disorders (Spiegel & Maldonado, 1999). As yet no universal definition or explanation of hypnosis has been postulated. Many theories, loosely classified under *state* and *nonstate* theories, have been advanced to explain hypnosis, but none of the theories has satisfactorily explained all the phenomena associated with. State theorists conceptualize hypnosis as a trance or altered state of consciousness (Barber, 1969, 1979), influenced by subjective traits and the states of the hypnotized person. The nonstate theorists purport a social, psychological explanation and maintain that there is nothing unique about hypnosis hypnosis; they argue that most hypnotic phenomena can occur without a hypnotic induction (Barber, 1969). These theorists focus on the social or relational aspects of the hypnotic interaction, and they emphasize the role of a variety of interactional forces, such as expectations and situational demands, in the production of hypnotic phenomena (Kirsch, 2000). These different formulations of hypnosis have broadened our understanding of the subject, but it is beyond the scope of this book to discuss the merits and controversies surrounding each theory (see Kallio & Revonsuo, 2003, for review, and rejoinder in the whole issue of *Contemporary Hypnosis*, 2005, 22 [1], pp. 1–55). From his review of the well-known theories of hypnosis 20 years ago, Rowley (1986, p. 23) concluded:

None of them seem to be able to deal adequately with all the phenomena which come under the general heading of hypnosis. This is perhaps not surprising given the tremendous variety of phenomena. Accordingly the theories have different ways of dealing with this variety. Some redefine hypnosis, e.g., Edmonston (1981). Others reinterpret subjective experience, e.g., Spanos (1982).... Despite these inadequacies, each of the theories has something to offer, a new conceptualization of the issues, a methodological approach, a new synthesis of the evidence. Of course, in one sense it is impossible to produce

3. Hypnosis and Hypnotherapy   43

a theory which is satisfactory to all researchers, for they are likely to have different criteria for evaluating theories.

Almost a decade later, Yapko (2003, p. 61) expressed similar opinions when addressing the complexity of the hypnotic concept:

With a subject as complex as hypnosis, the inadequacy of a single theory's ability to explain the broad range of responses on so many different dimensions of experience becomes glaringly apparent. The complexities of the subject of hypnosis, and even greater complexities of the human being capable of hypnosis, are so great that it seems highly improbable that a single theory can evolve to explain its origin and character.

Kallio and Revonsuo (2003) proposed a multilevel framework to explain the hypnotic phenomena, which is strongly endorsed by Spiegel (2005, p. 32), who commented that:

Multilevel explanations are an absolute necessity in understanding human mind/brain/body phenomena because we are both neurally based and social creatures who experience the world in mental phenomenal terms. To choose one of these domains as the complete explanatory context is to be by definition wrong.

Academics and experimentalists have generally endorsed nonstate, interpersonal, or multifactorial views of hypnosis, whereas clinicians have tended to adopt state, intrapersonal, or single views of hypnosis, particularly the neodissociation theory of hypnosis, described here. Proponents of both camps, however, agree that hypnotic suggestions can produce altered states, and that some subject variables can influence the hypnotic performance. The important subject variables include cooperation (Spanos & Barber, 1974), expectations (Barber, 1984, 1999), motivation (Araoz, 1981, 1985), and level of involvement in suggestion-related thoughts and images (Erickson & Rossi, 1979; Spanos & Barber, 1974). Kirsch (2005), a well-known nonstate or sociocognitive theorist, emphasizes that both state and nonstate theorists agree that hypnotic suggestions can produce altered states such as amnesia, analgesia, involuntariness, and others, although there is disagreement about whether these altered experiences depend on the prior induction of a trance state. To clinicians, who are mainly concerned with reducing a patient's distress, the debate whether trance exists or does not exists, or whether trance-induction is necessary or not necessary, although interesting, is not considered paramount. What is important in the clinical context is the skilful negotiation of variables to maximize therapeutic gains. To a clinician, hypnosis denotes:

An interaction between two people characterized by a number of inter- and intra-personal processes of which the "essence of hypnosis" only forms a part, if indeed it is present at all. These processes, which are not independent of one another (and which may apply to the behavior [sic] and experience of both the subject and the hypnotist) include the following: selective attention, imagination, expectancy, social conformity, compliancy, role-playing, attribution, usually though not necessarily, relaxation, rapport, suggestion, and hypnotic or trance experience. (Heap, 1988, p. 3)

Clinicians emphasize the subjectivity of hypnosis and recognize that hypnotic techniques must be individualized for each patient. This can involve drawing on techniques from more than one theoretical model. The treatment approach described in this book adopts different therapeutic techniques, derived from diverse theoretical conceptualizations. Golden, Dowd, and Friedberg (1987) describe this approach as *technical eclecticism*. Using this approach, the clinician, in order to maximize therapeutic effects, borrows techniques freely from diverse therapeutic approaches without necessarily accepting the theories from which the techniques were derived.

The neodissociation theory of hypnosis continues to be a dominant contemporary theory of hypnosis. It has inspired extensive research, and it provides a rationale for clinical work (Kihlstrom, 2003; Lynn & Kirsch, 2006). It also forms part of the integrated conceptualization of depression proposed in Chapter 4. The focus on the neodissociation theory here is not meant to discredit the contributions made by other competing or completing theories of hypnosis. In fact, the clinical approaches to the treatment of depression described in this book actively utilize techniques proposed by many other theories of hypnosis to maximize therapeutic gains.

## Neodissociation Theory of Hypnosis

Although controversial, Hilgard's (1973, 1974, 1977) neodissociation conceptualization of hypnosis is one of the most influential theories of hypnosis, both from an experimental and clinical standpoint. Hilgard describes hypnosis and other related phenomena such as fugues, possession states, multiple personality, and the like in terms of *dissociation* or *divided consciousness*. West (1967) defines dissociation as a psychological process in which information (incoming, stored, or outgoing) is actively deflected from integration with its usual or expected associations. This produces alterations in thoughts, feelings, or actions so that, for a period, certain information is not associated or integrated with other information in the usual or logical way. West regards such an experience to be either normal or pathological. Janet's early research (1907) established a close relationship between hypnosis and dissociation. Janet (1889) put forward the view that systems of ideas can become split off from the main personality and exist as an unconscious subordinated personality, capable of becoming conscious through hypnosis. The theory was applied to hypnosis and various other normal and pathological states such as automatism, amnesia, fugues, and multiple personality. Hilgard, by deriving ideas and concepts from information processing, selective attention, brain functioning, and the cognitive model of consciousness, reformulated the theory in contemporary terms and called it *neodissociation theory*. In Hilgard's reformulation, dissociation is seen as an extension of normal cognitive functioning. He posited that, during ordinary consciousness, information is processed on a number of levels by a hierarchy of cognitive operations and controls. Ordinarily, these operations are integrated, but during hypnosis or dissociation, the integration decreases, and certain aspects of experiences may not be available to consciousness. Dissociation or hypnotic involvement is seen as a cognitive process on a continuum ranging from minor or limited to profound and widespread. Hilgard also considered the role of the concept of *self* and *will* in his neodissociation theory. He maintained that hypnosis and other dissociative experiences all involve some degree of loss of voluntary control or *division of control.*

Hilgard's theory proposed that an individual possesses a number of cognitive systems, hierarchically arranged, with a central control structure (*executive ego*) and multiple superordinate and subordinate structures, each with its own input and output connections with the world. Although the executive ego is normally in control, the other structures can take over as a result of hypnotic-type suggestions or other similar procedures or situations. In other words, hypnosis or other similar procedures has the effect of dissociating these systems from one another, and some of these systems can be taken out of awareness or consciousness. A hypnotized individual may thus report feeling no pain, but the *hidden observer*—the name Hilgard gives to the cognitive system that is aware of what is going on—may report feelings of pain.

Hilgard (1977) has utilized experiments involving hypnotic analgesia and automatic writing to demonstrate this hidden observer effect. This effect can also be demonstrated by suggesting to the hypnotized subject that, when a prearranged signal such as the placing of the hypnotist's hand on the subject's shoulder is given, the hypnotist will be able to contact a "hidden part" of the psyche, unknown to the subject's present conscious "part." Hilgard claims that when this suggestion is given to responsive subjects, the hypnotist may then contact another system of control, which can speak, unaware of the normal "waking" or "hypnotized" part. These parts are not normally aware of each other, because they are separated by *amnesic barriers*. These amnesic barriers can sometimes break down partially or completely, causing incongruities. The automatic or involuntary nature of hypnotic responding can be easily explained by this process. For example, in automatic writing, the active part that is writing is dissociated or split from the conscious part, which is unaware that such activity is taking place. The hidden observer (or a covert cognitive system) is aware of the automatic writing. The hidden observer can also be accessed after the termination of hypnosis by providing posthypnotic instructions during hypnosis. Thus, the neodissociation theory proposes that, when a subject is hypnotized, only some of the cognitive systems are involved, while others remain unaffected. "Thus a person who experiences only a vague feeling of relaxation has only a very few low level cognitive systems affected. A person who experiences arm levitation and analgesia has many more cognitive systems affected" (Rowley, 1986, p. 16). Dissociation can be externally induced, self-induced, or it can occur spontaneously.

Hilgard's attempts to link hypnosis with consciousness seem intuitive and logical. With the recent upturn of interest in consciousness as an area of scientific study in affective and cognitive neuroscience (e.g., Gazzaniga, 2000; Mesulam, 2000; Zeman, 2001), the relationship between consciousness and hypnosis is likely to be further clarified. Some striking parallels have already been observed in the mental processes involved in dreaming and hypnosis. For example, Llinas and Pare (1991) observed dissociations between the specific and nonspecific thalamocortical systems underpinning dreaming, implying that a state of hyperattentiveness to intrinsic activity can occur without registering sensory input. Similarly, Furster (1995), in dreaming, observed a dissociation between context and sensory input and the cognitive features of dreaming including altered sense of time, absence of temporality, lack of guiding reality and critical judgment, anchoring in personal experience, and affective coloring. These findings led Gruzelier (1998, p. 18) to draw parallels between hypnosis and altered state of consciousness:

> The fragmented networks activated in the dream seem to lack the associative links to a time frame, anchored as they are in the present, without time tags and references. This could equally be a description of the hypnotic state as high susceptibles experience it.

Hilgard's neodissociation theory of hypnosis is, however, incomplete. Although he proposed cognitive structures, he gave little information about what happens inside them. It is also unclear how many cognitive systems a person possesses, and how many of these are engaged in hypnosis. Moreover, the neodissociation theory has been criticized for ignoring the role of social compliance factors. However, some followers of Hilgard have addressed the role of social compliance in hypnosis. For example, Nadon, Laurence, and Perry (1991) have proposed an interactionist approach in which both cognitive and social factors play a part.

The scientific validity of the hidden observer phenomenon also has been challenged. Although Hilgard (1977) and Watkins and Watkins (1979) have provided experimental evidence for the presence of the hidden observer (see Hilgard, 1977), the studies and interpretation of the hidden observer have been questioned by sociocognitive theorists. Spanos (1986, 1991; Spanos & Coe, 1992) has been the most vocal critic of the hidden observer phenomenon. In several studies, Spanos and his colleagues demonstrated that the reports of the hidden observer varied as a function of the explicitness of instructions that the subjects received about the nature of the hidden observer. For example, Spanos and Hewitt (1980) obtained reports of more or less hidden pain as a function of whether the subjects were told that their hidden parts would be either more aware or less aware of the actual amount of pain. Such findings led Spanos and Coe (1992) to conclude that the hidden observer phenomenon is not an intrinsic characteristic of hypnosis, but a social artifact shaped by a subject's expectancies and situational demand characteristics. One study (Spanos, Radtke, & Bertrand, 1984) thus manipulated the instructions to produce two hidden observers, one sorting memories of abstract words and the other storing memories of concrete words. This led Lynn and Kirsch (2006) to argue that the hidden observer is implicitly or explicitly suggested by the hypnotist; hence they dubbed the hidden observer phenomenon the *flexible observer*.

The fact that the hidden observer reports vary with instructions does not disprove the neodissociation theory of hypnosis. Khilstrom and Barnier (2005) declare that it is the very nature of hypnosis for the hypnotized subject's behaviors and experiences to be influenced by the wording of suggestions and the subject's interpretations of them. Therefore, studies supporting the hypothesis that covert reports are influenced by suggestions are not evidence that the hidden observer is a methodological artifact or not a reflection of the divided consciousness. Khilstrom and Barnier (2005) point out that researchers, "with their own areas of interest and expertise, will naturally emphasize one or the other aspect of hypnosis in their work. But . . . a proper understanding of hypnosis will only come from taking the hypnotic subject's experience seriously and seeking to understand how that experience emerges from the interaction of cognitive and social processes" (p. 149). Naish (2005) went even further, stating that the hypnotized person's *experience* should be the main subject of research and not his behavior. He contends that hypnosis research should be directed at elucidating the mechanisms that bring about the hypnotic experience, not extrapolating from simulation studies. He argues that studying simulators has little to contribute to the understanding of the hypnotic phenomenon, because simulators do not share their experience with the hypnotized person. He proposes that the role of simulators should be confined to studies involving spontaneous, nonsuggested hypnotic behavior. Naish believes it is perverse to ignore the genuine experiences and associated cortical changes occurring in hypnotized subjects and to simply confine the investigation to the social context of the experiment. For example, Szechtman, Woody, Bowers, and Nahmias (1998), in their brain-mapping studies, demonstrated that while highly hypnotizable subjects claimed to be experiencing hallucinations, the observed brain activity was extremely like that resulting from true sensory stimulation. Similarly, Kosslyn, Thompson, Constantini-Ferrando, Alpert, and Spiegel (2000) showed that hypnotized individuals cortically responded to suggested experiences (colors) rather than to the actual stimuli in measurable ways. Gruzelier (2005) believes sociocognitive theorists tend to ignore these findings due to their "lack of engagement with neuroscientific evidence," resulting from their "pedagogical background" and lack of appreciation of the reductionist levels of neuroscientific explanation. He believes, for example, that abundant neurophysiological and neurocognitive evidence supports the hypothesis that the anterior cingulated cortex and the left dorsolateral prefrontal cortex are involved in hypnotic analgesia. He laments that sociocognitive theorists continue to turn a blind eye to these findings, expressing concern that "while it is one thing to make the admission of a lack of understanding, it is quite unscientific to opine that there is no evidence for an ASC perspective, and to go on to attribute hypnosis to purely psychological constructs" (p. 4). Gruzelier (2005) believes the field of hypnosis can be unified through active collaboration between scientists with neurophysiological and social orientations.

## Altered State of Consciousness

Ludwig (1966) defined altered state of consciousness (ASC) as an altered state according to subjective experience and altered psychological functioning. According to Ludwig, alteration in sensory input, physiological changes, and motor activity can produce an altered state in which "one's perception of an interaction with the external environment is different than the internal experience" (Brown & Fromm, 1986, p. 34). Tart (1975), to avoid the debate on whether hypnosis is a state or not a state from a clinical perspective, distinguishes among *discrete states of consciousness* (d-SOC), *discrete altered state of consciousness* (d-ASC), and *baseline states of consciousness* (b-SOC).

A discrete state of consciousness (d-SOC) is defined by Tart (1975) as "a unique, dynamic pattern or configuration of psychological structures." Although the components or subsystems of the psychological structures with a d-SOC can show some variation, as in the ordinary waking state, sleep, or dreaming, "the overall pattern, the overall system properties remain recognizably the same." A discrete altered state of consciousness (d-ASC) refers to a state that is different from some baseline consciousness, forming a new system with unique properties that have been generated as a restructuring of consciousness or reality. The word "altered" is purely a descriptive term, carrying no value. In this sense, hypnotic experience generates from internal construction of attitudes, values, motivations, and expectancies. In other words, a hypnotic experience or a d-ASC is a subjective experience resulting from the reconfiguration or repatterning of existing resources or cognitions. Baseline consciousness is stabilized by a number of processes, including dealing with the variability in the environment. Baseline consciousness is akin to the concept of *cohesive self*. Kohut (1977) describes the cohesive self as a mental and physical unit that has cohesiveness in space and continuity in time. The cognitive-dissociative model of depression described in Chapter 4 regards some types of depression to be akin to a d-ASC, produced by the configuration of the cognitive distortions.

According to Brown and Fromm (1986) and Rowley (1986), Hilgard's theory of hypnosis appears to meet Ludwig's and Tart's criteria for an altered state of consciousness. It is easy to conceive how a subject might report that she felt rather unusual if some of her cognitive systems were dissociated from one another. Hilgard (1974) also states that these systems may be affected by situations other than hypnotic induction, for example through fatigue, drug use, or music. Hypnosis as an altered state of consciousness has been described both theoretically and experientially (e.g., Fromm, 1977; Gill and Brenman, 1959; Hilgard, 1977; Orne, 1959; Shor, 1959) along the dimension of alteration in perception, cognition, awareness of one's surroundings, and absorption in an unusual experience. For example, Orne (1959) demonstrated the presence of "trance logic" and negative and positive hallucinations in highly hypnotized subjects, but not in unhypnotized subjects. The study of consciousness, unconscious processing, and ASC has generated substantial interest in the neurosciences, and Gruzelier (2005) believes this is likely to herald fresh approaches to the neuroscientific understanding of hypnosis. For example, the Altered States of Consciousness research consortium was formed in Germany in 1998 to study the psychobiology of ASC, utilizing the latest models and methods in cognitive neuroscience. This 6-year, funded research consortium reported on the fruits of its labors (Vaitl, Birbaumer, Gruzelier, et al., 2005, pp. 98–127). The

paper reviewed the psychological and neurobiological investiga-
tions of consciousness and concluded that different states of consciousness are influenced by compromised brain structure, transient changes in brain dynamics such as disconnectivity, and
changes in neurochemical and metabolic processes. As regards
hypnosis, the review stated that "studies suggest that hypnosis
affects integrative functions of the brain and induces an alteration or even breakdown between subunits within brain responsible for the formation of conscious experience" (p. 110). Gruzelier
(2005) believes the reawakening of interest in ASC in cognitive
neuroscience will offer new perspectives in the understanding of
ASC and will facilitate revisiting of old considerations in a fresh
way.

## STRENGTHS AND LIMITATIONS OF HYPNOTHERAPY

Because this book is a treatment manual, it would be inappropriate to review all the clinical applications of hypnosis. Instead,
the rest of this chapter focuses on discussing the strengths and
limitations of the application of hypnosis to psychotherapy.

### Limitations of Hypnosis

#### *Lacking Unique Theoretical Underpinnings*

Hypnotherapy does not provide a theory of personality or psychopathology. Thus, a theoretical framework for conceptualizing
treatment is lacking: The manner in which hypnotherapy produces therapeutic outcome is very often not determined. As a
rule, hypnotherapy tends to be used in a shotgun fashion, without giving adequate attention to the disorder being treated and
without stating how hypnotherapy per se will be used to alleviate
the symptoms (Wadden & Anderton, 1982).

#### *Overemphasis on Unconscious Factors*

Traditionally, hypnotherapy has been very much influenced by
psychodynamic theories of psychopathology. Under such influence, therapists have tended to overemphasize the importance
of unconscious factors in the etiologies of psychological and psychosomatic disorders. As a result, they have tended to underplay the role of conscious cognitions (e.g., attitudes, beliefs, fantasies, self-talk, and thinking) and overt behaviors, which can
also cause and maintain symptoms and maladaptive behaviors.
Moreover, within the psychodynamic framework, conscious and
symptomatic interventions are considered harmful. Some hyp-
noanalysts (e.g., Brenman & Gill, 1947; Fromm, 1984) have ar-
gued that permanent change will not occur unless the patient's
unconscious conflicts are uncovered and worked through. These
attitudes, although helpful to some patients, have hindered the
expansion and exploration of other models of etiology and intervention. Consequently hypnotherapy has not made much of an
impact with certain disorders. For example, these attitudes created the myth that hypnosis is harmful to depressed patients
(Hartland, 1971). Alladin (1989, 1994, 2006; Alladin & Heap,
1991); Yapko (1992, 2001) have demonstrated that when hypnotherapy is appropriately combined with cognitive therapy, it
can become a very effective treatment for clinical depression.

### Passivity in Therapy

Traditionally, the patient has taken a passive role in hypnotherapy. Often a patient is given posthypnotic suggestions or encouraged to do certain things but, as a rule, he is not actively involved in monitoring and restructuring thoughts, feelings, behaviors, and physiological responses.

### Hypnosis Is Not Therapy

Although indirectly therapeutic, hypnotic induction is not therapy. Hypnotherapy is mainly used as an adjunctive technique to therapy. Very often the adjunctive techniques used cannot be differentiated from other cognitive-behavioral interventions. Some hypnotherapists insist on calling these techniques hypnotherapy. Wadden and Anderton (1982) state "it is unclear from both a theoretical and practical standpoint what criteria are used to identify a treatment as uniquely hypnotic." Instead of defining a treatment as hypnotherapy simply by labeling it as such (Lazarus, 1973), it is more pragmatic to acknowledge the utilization and integration of nonhypnotic techniques. Such acknowledgment is likely to encourage the exploration and integration of other theories and techniques, thus expanding clinical skills and resources.

### Insufficient Provision of Insight

Most often, when hypnotherapy is used as a treatment modality, the patient is not provided with any explanation of the cause of the disorder, how hypnotherapy will help, or what the patient can do to reduce symptoms. Active participation from the patient should be encouraged, especially when treating such chronic psychological disorders as anxiety or depression.

### Symptoms Removal

To a large extent, hypnosis focuses on removing symptoms. Little attempts are made to teach and establish active coping skills. Even Ericksonian therapists, who talk of unconscious experiential learning, do not directly teach coping skills to their patients; they focus on symptom relief. In fact, some of these therapists believe direct intervention produces patient resistance. Traditionally, hypnotherapists have not actively addressed maladaptive cognitions and behaviors. In such chronic conditions as anxiety and depression, "insight-oriented methods based on persuasion, reasoning and re-education are necessary to achieve symptom alleviation" (Golden, et al., 1987, pp. 1–2) and "therapeutic results are more enduring if symptom amelioration includes the modification of thoughts, feelings, and behavior patterns that maintain the symptoms" (Golden, et al., 1987, p. 7).

### Negative Self-Hypnosis Not Addressed

Although hypnotherapists usually teach patients self-hypnosis, the influence of negative self-hypnosis (NSH) (Araoz, 1981) is not addressed. Routine self-hypnosis undertaken while uncognizant of the power of NSH can be easily countered by NSH. When teaching self-hypnosis, both patient and therapist should be aware of the powerful sabotaging effect of NSH.

### Hypotheses Lacking Support

Rarely, data are provided to support the hypotheses of why
hypnosis work. For example, the efficacy of hypnosis is often
attributed to either heightened expectancy (Lazarus, 1973), therapeutic effects of the trance state (Weitzenhoffer, 1963), or enhancement of bodily relaxation and visual imagery (Kroger &
Fezler, 1976), but the data are rarely provided to support these
conclusions.

### Strengths of Hypnosis

Despite some of the limitations mentioned, hypnosis has many
strengths, and it can be made even more powerful when combined
with cognitive and other therapies.

### Adds Leverage to Treatment

When used properly, hypnosis adds leverage to treatment and
shortens treatment time (Dengrove, 1973). These effects could be
partly related to the rapid and profound behavioral, emotional,
cognitive, and physiological changes brought on by hypnosis (De
Piano & Salzberg, 1981).

### Strong Placebo Effect

For the majority of patients, hypnosis acts as a strong placebo.
Lazarus (1973) and Spanos and Barber (1974, 1976) have provided evidence that hypnotic trance induction procedures are
beneficial for those patients who believe in their efficacy. The
sensitive therapist can create the right atmosphere to capitalize
on suggestibility and expectation effects to enhance therapeutic
gains (Erickson & Rossi, 1979).

### Breaking Resistance

Indirect hypnotic suggestions can be provided to break a patient's
resistance. Erickson (Erickson & Rossi, 1979) has devised various
paradoxical instructions to minimize a patient's resistance to suggestions. For example, an oppositional patient may be instructed
(paradoxically) to continue to resist, as a strategy to obtain compliance. Another Ericksonian strategy for reducing resistance is
to use pacing and leading. The therapist is *pacing* an individual
when suggestions match the patient's ongoing behavior and experiences. As the patient becomes receptive to pacing, the therapist
can *lead* and offer more directive suggestions. For example, the
therapist may pace the patient by suggesting "as you exhale" as
the patient exhales, then lead by adding "you will begin to relax"
(Golden, et al., 1987, p. 3).

### Therapeutic Alliance

Repeated hypnotic experiences foster a strong therapeutic alliance (Brown & Fromm, 1987). Skilful induction of positive experiences, especially when patients perceive them to be emerging
from their own inner resources, give patients greater confidence
in their own abilities and help to foster trust in the therapeutic
relationship.

### Rapid Transference

Because of greater access to fantasies, memories, and emotions during hypnotic induction, full-blown transference manifestations may occur very rapidly, often during the initial stage of hypnotherapy (Brown & Fromm, 1987). Such transference reinforces the therapeutic alliance.

### Relaxation Response

Hypnosis induces relaxation, which is effective in reducing anxiety, making it easier for patients to think about and discuss materials that they were previously too anxious to confront. Sometimes anxious and agitated patients are also unable to pinpoint their maladaptive thoughts and emotions. Once they close their eyes and relax, many of these same individuals appear to become more aware of their thoughts and feelings. Through relaxation, hypnosis also reduces distraction and maximizes the ability to concentrate, which potentiates learning of new materials.

### Divergent Thinking

Hypnosis facilitates divergent thinking by (a) maximizing awareness along several levels of brain functioning, (b) maximizing focus of attention and concentration, and (c) minimizing distraction and interference from other sources of stimuli (Tosi & Baisden, 1984). In other words, through divergent operations, the potential for learning alternatives is increased.

### Attention to Wider Experiences

Hypnosis provides a frame of mind in which attention can be directed to wider experience, such as feeling of warmth, feeling happy, and the like. These experiences are more successfully produced following ego-strengthening suggestions (Hartland, 1971).

### Engagement of Nondominant Hemisphere

Hypnosis provides direct entry into the cognitive processing of the right cerebral hemisphere (in right-handers), which accesses and organizes emotional and experiential information. Therefore, during cognitive hypnotherapy (see Chapter 10), a patient can be taught techniques of hemispheric engagement or disengagement.

### Access to Nonconsciousness Processes

Hypnosis allows access to psychological processes below the threshold of awareness, thus providing a means of restructuring nonconscious cognitions.

### Integration of Cortical Functioning

Hypnosis provides a vehicle whereby cortical and subcortical functioning can be accessed and integrated. Because the subcortex is the seat of emotions, access to it provides an entry to the organization of primitive emotions.

### Imagery Conditioning

Hypnosis provides a basis for imagery training and conditioning. When the patient is hypnotized, the power of imagination is increased, possibly because hypnosis, imagery, and affect are all mediated by the same right cerebral hemisphere (Ley & Freeman, 1984). Under hypnosis, imagery can be used for the following reasons: (a) systematic desensitization (in imagination patient rehearses coping with in vivo difficult situations); (b) restructuring of cognitive processes at various levels of awareness or consciousness; (c) exploration of the remote past; and (d) directing attention on positive experiences. According to Boutin (1978), the rationale for using hypnosis is that it intensifies imagery and cognitive restructuring.

### Dream Induction

Hypnosis can induce dreams and increase dream recall and understanding (Golden, et al., 1987). Dream induction provides another vehicle for uncovering nonconscious maladaptive thoughts, fantasies, feelings, and images.

### Expansion of Experience

Hypnosis provides a vehicle for exploring and expanding experience in the present, past, and future. Such strategies can enhance divergent thinking and facilitate the reconstruction of dysfunctional "realities."

### Moods Induction

Negative or positive moods can be easily induced under hypnosis. Therefore, patients can be taught, through rehearsal, strategies for controlling negative or inappropriate affects. Mood induction can also facilitate recall. Bower (1981) has provided evidence that certain materials can only be recalled when experiencing the coincident mood (mood-state–dependent memory). Bower's research into mood-state–dependent memory led him to propose the associative network theory, which states: (a) an emotion serves as a memory unit that can easily link up with coincident events, (b) activation of this emotion unit can aid in the retrieval of events associated with it, and (c) mood primes emotional themata for use in free association, fantasies, and perceptual categorization.

### Posthypnotic Suggestions

Hypnosis provides posthypnotic suggestions, which can be very powerful in altering problem behaviors, dysfunctional cognitions, and negative emotions. Often, posthypnotic suggestions are used to shape behavior. Barrios (1973) regards posthypnotic suggestion to be a form of "higher-order conditioning," which functions as positive or negative reinforcement to increase or decrease the probability of desired or undesired behaviors, respectively. Clarke and Jackson (1983) have utilized posthypnotic suggestions to enhance the effect of in vivo exposure among agoraphobics.

### Positive Self-Hypnosis

Self-hypnosis training can be enhanced by heterohypnotic induction and posthypnotic suggestions. Most of the techniques mentioned here can be practiced under self-hypnosis, thus fostering positive self-hypnosis by deflecting preoccupation away from negative self-suggestions.

### Perception of Self-Efficacy

Bandura (1977) believes the expectation of self-efficacy is central to all forms of therapeutic change. Positive hypnotic experience, coupled with the belief that one has the ability to experience hypnosis and use hypnosis to alter symptoms, gives one an expectancy of self-efficacy, which can enhance treatment outcome.

### Easy Integration

Hypnosis provides a broad range of short-term techniques that can be easily integrated as an adjunct with many forms of therapy, for example, with behavior therapy, cognitive therapy, developmental therapy, psychodynamic therapy, supportive therapy, and others. Since hypnosis itself is not a therapy, the specific treatment effects will be contingent on the therapeutic approach with which it is integrated. Nevertheless, the hypnotic relationship can enhance the efficacy of therapy when hypnosis is used as an adjunct to a particular form of therapy (Brown & Fromm, 1987).

### SUMMARY

This chapter reviewed the neodissociation theory of hypnosis as it form an integral part of the cognitive-dissociative model of depression described in Chapter 4. The review clearly indicated that a perfect and complete theory of hypnosis is lacking. As Rowley (1986), Spiegel (2005), and Yapko (2003) indicated, hypnosis is a complex subject involving mind/brain/body phenomenon and, therefore, it will be impossible for a single theory to explain the broad range of human responses to it. Similarly, it is unlikely that a single physiological signature of hypnosis will be found. Because hypnosis involves a variety of phenomenological experience, various physiological underpinnings are bound to exist. Although intense debate exists about the nature of hypnosis between the state and nonstate theorists, there is agreement that hypnotic suggestions can produce altered states such as amnesia, analgesia, involuntariness, and the like. To clinicians, who are mainly concerned with reducing a patient's distress, the debate whether trance exist or does not exist, or whether trance-induction is necessary or not necessary is not considered paramount. What is important in the clinical context is the skilful negotiation of the patient's and technique's variables to maximize therapeutic gains. The chapter also highlighted the strengths and the limitations of hypnotherapy. The strengths of CBT and hypnotherapy can be combined to form a powerful treatment approach for depression, which is described in Part III of the book.

### REFERENCES

Alladin, A. (1989). Cognitive hypnotherapy for depression. In D. Waxman, D. Pederson, I. Wilkie & P. Mellett (Eds.), *Hypnosis: The 4th European congress at Oxford* (pp. 175–182). London: Whurr Publishers.

Alladin, A. (1994). Cognitive hypnotherapy with depression. *Journal of Cognitive Psychotherapy: An International Quarterly*, 8(4), 275–288.

Alladin, A. (2006). Cognitive hypnotherapy for treating depression. In R. Chapman (Ed.), *The clinical use of hypnosis in cognitive behavior therapy: A practitioner's casebook* (pp. 139–187). New York: Springer Publishing Company.

Alladin, A., & Heap, M. (1991). Hypnosis and depression. In M. Heap & W. Dryden (Eds.), *Hypnotherapy: A handbook* (pp. 49–67). Open University Press.

Araoz, D.L. (1981). Negative self-hypnosis. *Journal of Contemporary Psychotherapy*, 12, 45–52.

Araoz, D.L. (1985). *The new hypnosis*. New York: Brunner/Mazel.

Bandura, A. (1977). Self-efficacy: Toward a unifying theory of behavioral change. *Psychological Review*, 84, 191–215.

Barber, T.X. (1969). *Hypnosis: A scientific approach*. New York: Van Nostrand Reinhold.

Barber, T.X. (1979). Suggested ("hypnotic") behavior: The trance paradigm versus an alternative paradigm. In E. Fromm & R.E. Shor (Eds.), *Hypnosis: Developments in research and new perspectives* (2nd ed.). New York: Aldine.

Barber, T.X. (1984). Changing "unchangeable" bodily processes by (hypnotic) suggestions: A new look at hypnosis, cognitions, imagining, and the mind-body problem. In A.A. Sheikh (Ed.), *Imagination and healing* (pp. 69–127). Farmingdale, NY: Baywood.

Barber, T.X. (1999). A comprehensive three-dimensional theory of hypnosis. In I. Kirsch, A. Capafons, E. Cardena-Buelna, & S. Amigo (Eds.), *Clinical hypnosis and self-regulation: Cognitive-behavioral perspective* (pp. 21–48). Washington, DC: American Psychological Association.

Barrios, A.A. (1973). Posthypnotic suggestion in high-order conditioning: A methodological and experimental analysis. *International Journal of Clinical and Experimental Hypnosis*, 21, 32–50.

Boutin, G. (1978). The treatment of test anxiety by rational stage directed hypnotherapy. *American Journal of Clinical Hypnosis*, 21, 52–57.

Bower, G.H. (1981). Mood and memory. *American Psychologist*, 36, 129–148.

Brenman, M., & Gill, M.M. (1947). *Hypnotherapy: A survey of the literature*. Oxford, England, International Universities Press.

Brown, P.D., & Fromm, E. (1986). *Hypnotherapy and hypnoanalysis*. Hillsdale, NJ: Erlbaum.

Clarke, J.C., & Jackson, J.A. (1983). *Hypnosis and behavior therapy: The treatment of anxiety and phobias*. New York: Springer.

Dengrove, E. (1973). The use of hypnosis in behavior therapy. *International Journal of Clinical and Experimental Hypnosis*, 21, 13–17.

DePiano, F.A., & Salzberg, H.C. (1981). Hypnosis as an aid to recall of meaningful information presented under three types of arousal. *International Journal of Clinical and Experimental Hypnosis*, 29, 283–400.

Erickson, M.H., & Rossi, E. (1979). *Hypnotherapy: An exploratory casebook*. New York: Irvington.

Fromm, E. (1977). An ego-psychological theory for altered states of consciousness. *International Journal of Clinical and Experimental Psychology*, 25, 373–387.

Fromm, E. (1984). Theory and practice of hypnoanalysis. In W.C. Wester & A. Smith (Eds.), *Clinical hypnosis: A multidisciplinary approach* (pp. 142–154). New York: Lippincott.

Furster, J.M. (1995). *Memory in the cerebral cortex*. Cambridge: MIT Press.

Gazzaniga, M. (Ed.) (2000). *The new cognitive neurosciences*. Cambridge: MIT Press.

Gill, M.M., & Brenman, M. (1959). *Hypnosis and related states: Psychoanalytic studies in regression*. New York: International Universities Press.

Golden, W.L., Dowd, E.T., & Friedberg, F. (1987). *Hypnotherapy: A modern approach*. New York: Pergamon.

Gruzelier, J. (1998). A working model of the neurophysiology of hypnosis: A review of the evidence. *Contemporary Hypnosis*, 15, 3–21.

Gruzelier, J. (2005). Altered states of consciousness and hypnosis in the twenty-first century. *Contemporary Hypnosis*, 22, 1–7.

Hartland, J. (1971). *Medical and dental hypnosis and its clinical applications* (2nd ed.). London: Bailliere Tindall.

Heap, M. (Ed.) (1988). *Hypnosis: Current clinical, experimental and forensic practices*. London: Croom Helm.

Hilgard, E.R. (1973). The domain of hypnosis: With some comments on alternate paradigms. *American Psychologist*, 28, 972–982.

Hilgard, E.R. (1974). Toward a neo-dissociation theory: Multiple cognitive controls in human functioning. *Perspectives in Biology and Medicine*, 17, 301–316.

Hilgard, E.R. (1977). Divided consciousness: Multiple controls in human thought and action. New York: John Wiley & Sons.

Janet, P. (1889). *L' Automatisme psychologique*. Paris: Felix Alcan.

Janet, P. (1907). *The major symptoms of hysteria*. New York: Macmillan.

Kallio, S., & Revonsuo, A. (2003). Hypnotic phenomena and altered states of consciousness: A multilevel framework of description and explanation. *Contemporary Hypnosis*, 20, 111–164.

Kihlstrom, J.F. (2003). The fox, the hedgehog, and hypnosis. *International Journal of Clinical and Experimental Hypnosis*, 51, 166–189.

Kihlstrom, J.F., & Barnier, A.J. (2005). The hidden observer: A straw horse, undeservedly flogged. *Contemporary Hypnosis*, 22, 144–151.

Kirsch, I. (2000). The response set theory of hypnosis. *American Journal of Clinical Hypnosis*, 42, 3–4, 274–293.

Kirsch, I. (2005). Empirical resolution of the altered state debate. *Contemporary Hypnosis*, 22, 18– 23.

Kohut, H. (1977). *The restoration of the self*. New York: International Universities.

Kosslyn, S.M., Thompson, W.L., Costantini-Ferrando, M.F., Alpert, N.M., & Spiegel, D. (2000). Hypnotic visual illusion alters color processing in the brain. *American Journal of Psychiatry*, 157, 1279–1284.

Kroger, W.S., & Fezler, W.D. (1976). *Hypnosis and behavior modification: Imagery conditioning*. Philadelphia: J.B. Lippincott Company.

Lazarus, A.A. (1973). "Hypnosis" as a facilitator in behavior therapy. *International Journal of Clinical and Experimental Hypnosis*, 6, 83–89.

Ley, R.G., & Freeman, R.J. (1984). Imagery, cerebral laterality, and the healing process. In A.A. Sheikh (Ed.), *Imagination and healing* (pp. 51–68). New York: Baywood.

Llinas, R.R., & Pare, D. (1991). Of dreaming and wakefulness. *Neuroscience*, 44, 521–535.

Ludwig, A.M. (1966). Altered states of consciousness. In C.T. Tart (Ed.), *Altered states of consciousness* (pp. 9–22). New York: John Wiley & Sons, Inc.

Lynn, S.J., & Kirsch, I. (2006). *Essentials of clinical hypnosis: An evidence-based approach*. Washington, DC: American Psychological Association.

Mesulam, M.M. (Ed.) (2000). Principles of behavioral and cognitive neurology. Oxford: Oxford University Press.

Nadon, R., Laurence, J.R., & Perry, C. (1991). The two disciplines of scientific hypnosis: A synergistic model: In S.J. Lynn & J.W. Rhue (Eds.), *Theories of hypnosis: Current models and perspectives* (pp. 485–519). New York: Guilford Press.

Naish, P. (2005). Detecting hypnotically altered states of consciousness. *Contemporary Hypnosis*, 22, 24–30.

Orne, M.T. (1959). The nature of hypnosis: Artifact and essence. *Journal of Abnormal Psychology*, 58, 277–299.

Rowley, D.T. (1986). *Hypnosis and hypnotherapy*. London: Croom Helm.

Shor, R.E. (1959). Hypnosis and the concept of the generalized reality-orientation. *American Journal of Psychotherapy*, 13, 582–602.

Spanos, N.P. (1986). Hypnotic behavior: A social-psychological interpretation of amnesia, analgesia and "trance logic." *Behavioral and Brain Sciences*, 9, 449–502.

Spanos, N.P. (1991). A sociocognitive approach to hypnosis. In S.J. Lynn & J.W. Rhue (Eds.), *Theories of hypnosis: Current models and perspectives* (pp. 324–361). New York: Guilford.

Spanos, N.P., & Barber, T.X. (1974). Toward a convergence in hypnosis research. *American Psychologist*, 29, 500–511.

Spanos, N.P., & Barber, T.X. (1976). Behavior modification and hypnosis. In M. Hersen, R.M. Eisler, & P.M. Miller (Eds.), *Progress in behavior modification*. New York: Academic.

Spanos, N.P., & Coe, W.C. (1992). A social psychological approach to hypnosis. In E. Fromm & M.R. Nash (Eds.), *Contemporary hypnosis research* (pp. 102–130). New York: Guilford.

Spanos, N.P., & Hewitt, E.C. (1980). The hidden observer in hypnotic analgesia: Discovery or experimental creation? *Journal of Personality and Social Psychology*, 39, 1201–1214.

Spanos, N.P., Radtke, H.L., & Bertrand, L.D. (1984). Hypnotic amnesia as a strategic enactment: Breaching amnesia in highly hypnotizable subjects. *Journal of Personality and Social Psychology*, 47, 1155–1169.

Spiegel, D. (2005). Multileveling the playing field: Altering our state of consciousness to understand hypnosis. *Contemporary Hypnosis*, 22, 31–33.

Spiegel, D., & Maldonado, J.R. (1999). Hypnosis. In R.E. Hales, S.C. Yudofsky, & J.A. Talbot (Eds.), *Textbook of psychiatry* (3rd ed.) (pp. 1243–1274). Washington, DC: American Psychiatric Press.

Szechtman, H., Woody, E., Bowers, K.S., & Nahmias, C. (1998). Where the imaginal appears real: A positron emission tomography study of auditory hallucinations. *Proceedings of the National Academy of Sciences*, 95, 1956–1960.

Tart, C. (1975). *States of consciousness*. New York: Dutton.

Tosi, D.J., & Baisden, B.S. (1984). Cognitive-experiential therapy and hypnosis. In W.C. Wester & A.H. Smith (Eds.), *Clinical hypnosis: A multidisciplinary approach* (pp. 155–178). New York: J.B. Lippincott.

Vaitl, D., Birbaumer, N., Gruzelier, J., Jamieson, G., Kotchoubey, B., Kubler, A., et al. (2005). Psychobiology of altered states of consciousness. *Psychology Bulletin*, 131, 98–127.

Wadden, T.A., & Anderton, C.H. (1982). The clinical use of hypnosis. *Psychological Bulletin*, 91, 215–243.

Watkins, J.G., & Watkins, H.H. (1979). Ego sates and hidden observers. *Journal of Altered States of Consciousness*, 5, 3–18.

Weitzenhoffer, A.M. (1963). *Hypnotism: An objective study in suggestibility*. New York: John Wiley & Sons.

West, L.J. (1967). Dissociative reaction. In A.M. Freedman & H.I. Kaplan (Eds.), *Comprehensive textbook of psychiatry*. Philadelphia: Williams & Wilkins Co.

Yapko, M.D. (1992). *Hypnosis and the treatment of depressions: Strategies for change*. New York: Brunner-Mazel.

Yapko, M.D. (2001). *Treating depression with hypnosis: Integrating cognitive-behavioral and strategic approaches*. New York: Brunner-Routledge.

Yapko, M.D. (2003). *Trancework: An introduction to the practice of clinical hypnosis* (3rd ed.) New York: Brunner-Routledge.

Zeman, A. (2001). Consciousness. *Brain*, 124, 1263–1289.

# II

# A New Working Model of Depression

# 4

# Circular Feedback Model
# of Depression

After reviewing the relative strengths and limitations of CBT and hypnotherapy, it would appear clinically intuitive to combine the strengths of the two treatments. Such integration not only compensates for the shortcomings of each treatment, but also shapes clinical practice guidelines. This chapter describes a working model of depression referred as the *circular feedback model of depression* (CFMD) that provides the theoretical and empirical rationale for integrating CBT with hypnotherapy in the management of depression. This is a biopsychosocial model of depression, emphasizing the circular nature of the disorder. An important element of circularity is that it encourages intervention simultaneously at multiple levels. The major contribution of the model—beyond its value as an organizational tool—is its emphasis on functional autonomy and circular causality, so that factors such as cognitive distortions, negative ruminations, distressed relationships, adverse life events, and neurochemical changes are seen as both symptoms and causes at the same time. Before describing CFMD, the literature pertaining to hypnotherapy for depression is first reviewed.

## HYPNOTHERAPY FOR DEPRESSION

Despite the fact that depression is an urgent and widespread problem, hypnotherapy has not been widely used in the management of clinical depression. I (2006) believe this may be due to the erroneous belief among some writers and clinicians that hypnotherapy can exacerbate suicidal behaviors in depressed patients. For example, Hartland (1971) warned that "hypnosis should *never* be used in depressional states in which suicidal impulses are present unless the patient is an in-patient under hospital supervision" (p. 335; emphasis in original text). More recently, however, clinicians have proposed that hypnotherapy, when it forms part of a multimodal treatment approach, is not contraindicated in either inpatient or outpatient depressed patients (e.g., Alladin, 2006; Alladin & Heap, 1991; Yapko, 1992, 2001). For example, Yapko (1992) utilizes hypnotherapy to reduce symptoms of hopelessness, which is a predictor of suicidal behavior, in the early stages of his comprehensive approach to psychotherapy for depression. The bulk of the published literature on the application of hypnosis in the management of depression has consisted of case reports (Burrows & Boughton, 2001). Because of the great deal of variation in the techniques reported in these cases, it is difficult to compare directly the various methods employed by individual therapists in the management of depression.

Nevertheless, a growing body of research evaluates the use of hypnotherapy with CBT in the treatment of various psychological disorders, although not specifically with depression. Schoenberger (2000), from her review of the empirical status of the use of hypnotherapy in conjunction with CBT, concluded that the existing studies demonstrate substantial benefits from the addition of hypnotherapy to cognitive-behavioral techniques. Similarly, Kirsch, Montgomery, and Sapirstein (1995), from their meta-analysis of 18 studies comparing CBT with the same treatment supplemented by hypnotherapy, found the mean effect size to be larger than the nonhypnotic treatment. The authors concluded that hypnotherapy was significantly superior to nonhypnotic treatment. Encouraged by these findings, several writers (e.g., Golden, Dowd, & Friedberg, 1987; Tosi & Baisden, 1984; Yapko, 2001) have described the integration of CBT and hypnotherapy with depression. Research undertaken by my associates and I (Alladin, 1989, 1992, 1994, 2006; Alladin & Heap, 1991) has provided a theoretical rationale and solid empirical foundation for combining these two treatment approaches. This is in marked contrast to the work of other researchers: Yapko (2001) remarks, "Therapeutic efficacy research involving hypnosis specifically for depression has, to this point, been essentially nonexistent" (p. 7).

My working model of nonendogenous depression, CDMD, provides a theoretical framework for integrating cognitive and hypnotic techniques with depression. Research data (Alladin, 2005, 2006; Alladin & Alibhai, 2007) have demonstrated an increase in effect size when hypnotherapy is combined with CBT in the management of chronic depression. We (Alladin, 2005; Alladin & Alibhai, 2007) compared the effects of CBT with cognitive hypnotherapy in 98 chronically depressed patients. The results showed an additive effect for combining hypnotherapy with CBT. The study also met criteria for *probably efficacious* treatment for depression as outlined by the American Psychological Association (APA) Task Force (Chambless & Hollon, 1998), and it provides empirical validation for integrating hypnosis with CBT in the management of depression. The results of the study are discussed in greater detail under Effectiveness of Cognitive Hypnotherapy in Chapter 5. In this book, CDMD has been revised, refined, and renamed the *circular feedback model of depression* (CFMD).

## CIRCULAR FEEDBACK MODEL OF DEPRESSION

CFMD is conceptualized to emphasize the circular and biopsychosocial nature of depression and to elucidate the role of multiple factors that can trigger, exacerbate, or maintain the depressive affect. The model is not a new theory of depression or an attempt to explain the causes of depression. It is an extension of Beck's (1967) circular feedback model of depression, which was later elaborated on by Schultz (1978, 1984, 2003). This extended model combines cognitive and hypnotic paradigms, and it incorporates ideas and concepts from information processing, selective attention (cognitive distortion, rumination), brain functioning, adverse life experiences, and the neodissociation theory of

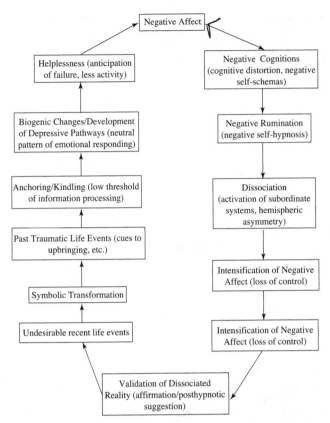

**Fig. 4.1. Circular feedback model of depression (CFMD) showing the constellation of 12 factors forming the depressive loop.**

hypnosis. It is referred as the circular feedback model because it consists of 12 interrelated components that form a circular feedback loop (Fig. 4.1). From the review of the theories of depression in Chapters 1 and 2, it is apparent that depression is related to a host of interacting processes in the domains of physiological processes (genes and hormones), psychological factors (negative beliefs, rumination, and social withdrawal), and social factors (life events and social support) that interact over time (Akiskal & McKinney, 1975; Gilbert, 2004). The number of components forming the loop and the position of each component in the loop is arbitrary. The 12 components forming the circular loop represent some of the major sets of factors identified from the literature that may influence the onset, course, and outcome of depression. Any one of these 12 components, singly or in concert with other components, can synergistically trigger, exacerbate, or maintain the depressive affect. Moreover, the interaction among these components is dynamic, ongoing, and reciprocal in nature.

This chapter describes the model, then presents an integrated approach to treatment based on the model. This treatment approach is called *cognitive hypnotherapy* (CH). CH is a structured program of therapy, described in Part III of the book, that utilizes hypnotherapeutic methods along with orthodox cognitive and behavioral procedures (Alladin & Heap, 1991) in the treatment of depression. The 12 components are described in detail below, and the relationships among these components that form the depressive loop is highlighted.

**Negative Affect and Negative Cognitions**

Because the model attaches significant importance to the interaction between affect and cognition, the logical starting point for describing the depressive loop is to start with affect, which appears at the top of the loop (Fig. 4.1). The CFMD proposed by Beck (1967) maintains the existence of a mutually reinforcing interaction between cognition and affect so that thought not only influences feelings, but feelings too can influence thought content (hence the bidirectional arrows between *Negative Affect* and *Negative Cognition* in Fig. 4.1). Also, congruent with the concepts of the "bicameral brain" (Jaynes, 1976) and unconscious information processing (e.g., LeDoux, 2000), it is maintained that either affect or cognition can independently starts the chain process of the feedback loop (Fig. 4.1). The intimate association between dysfunctional cognition and depressive affect is well documented in the literature (e.g., Haas & Fitzgibbon, 1989; Haaga, Dyck, & Ernst, 1991). An event (internal or external) can trigger a negative schema that, through cognitive rehearsal, can lead to dissociation.

**Negative Self-Hypnosis**

Individuals predisposed to depression not only focus on negative thoughts but also on negative imagery. Schultz (1978), Starker and Singer (1975), and Traynor (1974) have provided evidence that with increasing levels of depression, depressed patients tend to change the content of their fantasies and focus more on negative topics. Such focusing generates negative imagery and leads to the maintenance and exacerbation of the depressed mood that initially produced the negative thinking. Consequently, depressed patients are unable to change the negative content of their imagination. Moreover, Schultz (1978) found that depressed patients are unable to redirect their thinking and imagery away from their current problems; hence, the depressive mood is continually reinforced. In other words, the circular feedback cycle between cognition and affect repeats itself almost like a computer reverberating through an infinite loop (Schultz, 1978). This process is very similar to the concept of negative self-hypnosis (NSH) proposed by Araoz (1981, 1985) to explain the maintenance of emotional disorders.

The concept of NSH can be easily extended to explain the persistence of the depressive process. Because depressed patients (when depressed) tend to be actively involved in NSH, it is not surprising that they have little success in breaking the affective circular feedback loop. This explains Schultz's (1978) findings that depressed patients are unable to relieve depression through nondirected or passive imagery. In fact, such nondirected imagery led to a worsening of the depression. On the other hand, active or directed imagery (since this did not allow indulgence in active NSH) led to a reduction in depression. NSH, in the context of depression, can be conceptualized as a form of depressive rumination.

## Depressive Rumination

Depressive rumination is a common response to negative moods (Rippere, 1977). It can be crudely defined as persistent and recyclic depressive thinking (Papageorgiou & Wells, 2004). Rumination is not always negative. Research suggests rumination is a natural, normal phenomenon, providing us with a way of getting back on track with our goals (Papageorgiou & Wells, 1999). At times, however, rumination can be undesirable and counterproductive, thwarting individuals from goal attainment. In these instances, the ruminative state tends to persist. This is particularly noticeable among depressed patients. Nolen-Hoeksema and her colleagues have been instrumental in advancing our knowledge of ruminative thinking in depression. Nolen-Hoeksema (1991, 2004) proposed the *response styles theory of depression*, which conceptualizes rumination as repetitive and passive thinking about symptoms of depression and the possible causes and consequences of these symptoms. Several studies (see Papageorgiou & Wells, 2004) have provided evidence that depressed patients tend to ruminate for longer duration, exert little effort to problem-solve, express lower confidence in problem-solving, and have a greater orientation to the past. According to the response styles theory, depressive rumination exacerbates and prolongs symptoms of depression, and aggravates moderate symptoms of depression into major depressive episodes. Within the CFMD model, depressive rumination is conceptualized as a form cognitive distortion or NSH.

Nolen-Hoeksema (2004) has posited four mechanisms by which depressive rumination prolongs depression. First, rumination enhances the effects of depressed mood on cognitive distortions, thus potentiating negative appraisal of the current circumstances (based on memories activated by depressed mood). Second, rumination interferes with effective problem-solving by promoting pessimistic and fatalistic thinking. Third, rumination interferes with instrumental behavior. Finally, people who chronically ruminate lose social support, which in turn feeds on their depression. From their review of the large number of studies on ruminative responses to depressed mood, Lyubomirsky and Tkach (2004) demonstrated rumination to have negative consequences on thinking, motivation, concentration, problem-solving, instrumental behavior, and social support. Moreover, Nolen-Hoeksema (2000), using a community sample of 1,300 depressed adults, found rumination to be strongly related to the development of a mixed anxiety-depression syndrome. Content analyses of the ruminators' ruminations revealed that anxiety was related to uncertainty over whether one will be able to control one's environment, whereas depression was related to hopelessness about the future and negative evaluation of the self. In other words, ruminators may vacillate between anxiety and depression as their cognition vacillates between uncertainty and hopelessness. This process partially explains the comorbid relationship between anxiety and depression.

From this discussion it is evident that negative rumination is a potential risk factor for depression, and it plays an important part in the exacerbation and maintenance of the depressive affect. In this context, it is also not unreasonable to consider NSH as a form of negative rumination. Since the concept of rumination has been studied extensively, it is tempting to replace NSH with rumination. However, the concept of NSH is preserved in the model to encourage research on NSH and to emphasize the dissociative aspect of rumination. Studies of NSH in the context of depression are likely to provide further understanding on how attention is automatically directed toward negative self-relevant material to create a mental environment that is conducive to the intensification of negative affect and negative self-affirmations (negative posthypnotic suggestions). Studies of the relationship between NSH and depression are likely to provide insight into the phenomenological nature of the depressive state.

## Conceptualization of Depression as Dissociation

NSH can be regarded as a form of dissociation. According to Araoz (1981, 1985), NSH consists of nonconscious (automatic) rumination with negative statements and defeatist mental images that the person indulges in, encourages, and often works hard at fostering—while at the same time consciously wanting to get better. Araoz calls this NSH because it is composed of three hypnotic components: (i) noncritical thinking that becomes a negative activation of subconscious processes, (ii) active negative imagery, and (iii) powerful posthypnotic suggestions in the form of negative affirmations. I (1992) contend that, like hypnosis, unipolar nonendogenous depression also involves all three components. Such a process can be readily observed in depressed patients, who are constantly ruminating on their alleged negative personal attributes, which can be regarded as a form of self-hypnotic induction. Although not making reference to hypnosis or dissociation, Beck, Rush, Shaw, and Emery (1979, p. 13) state:

In milder depressions the patient is generally able to view his negative thoughts with some objectivity. As the depression worsens, his thinking becomes increasingly dominated by negative ideas, although there may be no logical connection between actual situations and his negative interpretations. . . . In the more severe states of depression, the patient's thinking may become completely dominated by the idiosyncratic schema: he is completely preoccupied with perseverative, repetitive negative thoughts and may find it enormously difficult to concentrate on external stimuli . . . or engage in voluntary mental activities. . . .

In such instances we infer that the idiosyncratic cognitive organization has become autonomous. The depressive cognitive organization may become so independent of external stimulation that the individual is unresponsive to changes in his immediate environment.

Because strong emotions narrow the focus of attention to affectively relevant events and exclude incidental stimuli

(Easterbrook, 1959), emotionally upset people, such as depressed patients, become poor learners (e.g., Beck, 1967); they are distracted away from alternative channels of information. During normal waking state, single-channel cognitive processing is normally involved (Shevrin & Dickman, 1980), but in such states as dream, intoxication, psychosis, multiple personality, and the like, the single-channel characteristic is not shared. Hilgard (1977) believes that multiple-channels (divided consciousness) may be involved in these states. Moreover, Hilgard (1977) takes the concept of "self" and "will" into consideration, and maintains that hypnosis and other dissociative experiences all involve some degree of loss of voluntary control, or a division of control. This is very noticeable in depressed patients, who report having very little self-esteem and have lost the will to do anything. Hilgard also talks about the central structure or the executive ego, which is normally in control, but that can be taken over by other subordinate structures as a result of hypnotic-type suggestions or other similar procedures or situations. In depression, the patient's constant negative rumination can easily induce negative self-hypnosis (dissociation), which in turn can strengthen subordinate cognitive structures or schemas. Once these subordinate systems have been established, they can develop a certain degree of autonomy via rumination or self-hypnosis. Hence, activities that are normally under control may go out of voluntary control (partly or completely); consequently, the associated experiences may go out of normal awareness. Such focusing also leads to an impoverished construction of reality (i.e., based on selective information processing), permitting continual reinforcement of the depressive feedback loop. Neisser (1967) regards such narrowing down and distortion of the environment by a few repetitive behaviors and self-attributions as characteristic of psychopathology. In other words, once depressed individuals are involved in the depressive loop, their cognitive distortions become automatic (dissociative), and hence they are unable to focus on alternative thinking and images not related to their current problems and negative life concerns. I (1992) propose that negative rumination in some depressed patients may lead to a state of partial or profound dissociation.

The circular feedback model, however, does not regard hypnosis or dissociation to be analogous to depression. Rather, it proposes that there are some commonalities in the style of cognitive processing and organization (depressive rumination) involved in the generation of the "state of hypnosis" and the "state of depression." Since it is possible to hypnotically induce transient and long-lasting negative or positive psychological and physiological changes, hypnosis provides a paradigm for studying and understanding how negative ruminations produce and intensify depressive affect. My research (1992) has highlighted the similarities and differences between hypnosis and depression, and makes note of the fundamental difference between the two states in terms of cognitive contents and control. The cognitive contents of hypnosis can be either negative or positive, and they can be easily altered (easily controlled), whereas the cognitive contents of depression are invariably negative and not easily changed (not easily controlled). A variety of evidence (for a review see Tomarken

& Keener, 1998) indicates that depressed individuals, because of the relative hypoactivity of their left frontal brain, demonstrate enhanced negative affective responses to emotion elicitors (e.g., depressive rumination, negative affect) that are more likely to be sustained over time. This is caused by a heightened access to cognitive or other processes that serve to sustain negative affective reactions and decreased access to processes that inhibit negative affect to promote the positive-affect–induced counter-regulation of negative affect. Although indirectly describing how NHS produces the phenomenological experience of the depressive affect, this divided consciousness may also be involved in unipolar depression.

## Cerebral Lateralization in Depression and Hypnosis

In this section, neuropsychophysiological correlates of emotion, depression, imagery, rumination, and hypnosis are briefly reviewed to identify the similarities and differences in the brain correlates among these states and to integrate this information in the development of treatment strategies.

A variety of evidence indicates a linkage between depression and specific patterns of frontal brain asymmetry. Unilateral brain lesions, unilateral hemispheric sedation, electroencephalographic (EEG) studies, positron emission tomography (PET), single photon emission tomography (SPECT), functional magnetic resonance imaging (fMRI), and biochemical studies indicate that unipolar depression is associated with decreased activation of left-hemisphere frontal brain regions relative to right-hemisphere frontal regions (for a review, see Tomarken & Keener, 1998; Davidson, Pizzagalli, & Nitschke, 2002; Mayberg, 2006). Of prime importance from these findings is that (a) the resting frontal brain asymmetry may be a trait marker for vulnerability to depression, and (b) relative left-frontal hyperactivation may be linked to decreased vulnerability to depression and to a self-enhancing cognitive style that may promote such decreased vulnerability. However, at this point it is not known why brain asymmetry is linked to depression. Davidson (see Davidson, Pizzagalli, & Mitschke, 2002) has invoked the *approach-withdrawal hypothesis* to account for the linkage between frontal brain asymmetry and depression.

According to the approach-withdrawal hypothesis, relative left-frontal activation is associated with heightened appetitive or incentive motivation, heightened responsivity to rewards or other positive stimuli, and greater contact with those features of the external environment that are rewarding or engaging. Relative right-frontal activation is associated with a protective-defensive tendency to withdraw from potentially threatening stimuli (e.g., novel ones) or to avoid such stimuli. Several empirical findings support the approach-withdrawal hypothesis. For example, Calkins, Fox, and Marshall (1996) showed that children who display behavioral inhibition or social reticence are more likely to demonstrate relative right-frontal activation. Such children tend to withdraw from novel stimuli, whereas uninhibited children tend to approach such stimuli. The approach-withdrawal hypothesis is also consistent with the evidence that frontal brain asymmetry is linked to depression or risk of depression (Henriques & Davidson, 1990). Henriques and Davidson (1990) purport that anhedonia and decreased reactivity to pleasurable stimuli linked with depression may reflect a deficit in a reward-oriented approach system. Studies also suggest the link between left-frontal hypoactivation in depression and a deficit in dopaminergic function (Ebert, Feistel, Kaschka, Barocka, & Pirner, 1994). However, it is notable that experimentally induced positive affect both facilitates delay of gratification (Fry, 1977) and induces left-frontal activation (e.g., Ekman, Davidson, & Friesen, 1990). These findings have implications for treatment. Positive affect induced by imagery or hypnotherapy can activate the left hemisphere and in turn promote goal-approach behaviors.

In the context of the present discussion, it should be pointed out that in normal individuals the hemispheres do not comprise two independent, distinctly different brains. There is overlap in the functions of the two, and most complex processing involves activation in both hemispheres. However, it is important to keep in mind that some well-established differences exist between the left and right hemispheres, and a consideration of these differences may help us develop theories about depression, hypnosis, and rumination. Neuropsychological studies of hypnosis and depression suggest some functional and structural similarities between the two states. Although the two cerebral hemispheres interact with each other, there is lateralized specialization in terms of information processing. The left or dominant hemisphere excels in verbal, logical, critical, and analytical perception and cognition, whereas the right or nondominant hemisphere is skilled in nonverbal, emotional, uncritical, and holistic apprehension of information (see Martin, Shrira, & Startup, 2004).

As discussed in Chapter 3, as yet no "brain signature" of hypnosis has been identified. Earlier neuropsychological models of hypnosis suggested an overall right-hemispheric involvement during hypnosis (e.g., Graham, 1977). There is no evidence that individuals rely on only one hemisphere for thinking or carrying out a cognitive task. Moreover, low- and high-hypnotizable individuals demonstrate differential hemispheric patterns of activity. Recent research demonstrates that most cognitive activity may be broken down into componential stages, which then correlate with activation of different parts of the brain (Crawford & Gruzelier, 1992). Gruzelier (2000) asserts, based on accumulating evidence, that during the sequential hypnotic induction, an alteration occurs in the relationship among the various anterior–posterior, left–right, and cortical–subcortical axes of brain functional organization. This led Gruzelier to propose a three-stage model of the neuropsychophysiology of hypnosis (see Yapko, 2003 for summary). The first stage involves increased frontal lobe activity in the left hemisphere, congruent with the attention directed to the hypnotist's voice. In the second stage, as the person being hypnotized "lets go," concomitant inhibition occurs in the frontolimbic process. In the third stage, the hypnotized person is very absorbed; hence there is a "redistribution of functional activity and an augmentation of posterior cortical activity, particularly of the right hemisphere" (p. 2). Based on these observations,

Gruzelier recommends the use of traditional methods of hypnotic induction. According to Gruzelier, these methods follow the sequence of sensory fixation, relaxation, sleepiness, concentrated attention, suggestions, and so on, in an attempt to follow a logical neurophysiological sequence: "the engaging of anterior left-sided attentional mechanisms, which once engaged can be suppressed, which in turn allows selective inhibition of frontal functions permitting cardinal features of the hypnotic experience such as automaticity and involuntariness to take place" (p. 55).

De Pascalis (1999) has also observed that, early in the hypnotic induction process, the left hemisphere is more active but, as the induction progresses, the left hemisphere's activity is inhibited. Spiegel and Spiegel (2004) believe accumulating evidence shows that hypnosis involves alteration in the anterior attentional system, especially in the anterior cingulate gyrus, and that hypnotic alteration of perception results in congruent changes in brain electrical activity and blood flow in the salient sensory cortex. The fact that hypnotized individuals exhibit hemispheric specificity, left or right, depending on task demands, has significant therapeutic implication for depression. Crawford & Gruzelier (1992, pp. 228–229) state:

Numerous studies have demonstrated that those individuals who have the ability to refocus their attention and shift cognitive strategies when given a hypnotic induction are generally also capable of vivid imagination, holistic thinking, extremely focused and sustained attention, and absorption in imaginative activities ... also of disattending to task-irrelevant environmental stimuli ... demonstrate greater abilities ... in shifting from one strategy to another and from one alternate state of awareness to another—an ability we have referred to as "cognitive flexibility."

The ability to "disattend" to irrelevant stimuli (to habituate) provides a major clue as to what contributes to the development of dissociative behavior. More central to hypnosis is the inhibition of anterior frontal lobe functions. There is good agreement on primary right-hemispheric involvement in the hypnotic trance per se. Sheehan (1992) has described several strategies for facilitating hypnotic subjects to respond to hypnotic suggestions and realize positive hypnotic experience. Some of these strategies are integrated with the various hypnotherapeutic strategies described in Chapters 9, 10, and 11.

Some commonalities exist among depression, hypnosis, and rumination in terms of cerebral hemisphere specialization. Rumination is an instance of the *Zeigarnik effect* (Martin, Shrira, & Startup, 2004). Zeigarnik (1938) demonstrated that information related to incomplete tasks tends to remain in memory longer than information related to completed tasks. From the goal-progress view, rumination is essentially the tendency to think recurrently about important, higher-order goals that have not yet been attained. Rumination is instigated not just by failure to attain a goal, however, but also by failure to progress toward a goal at a rate that matches the individual's standard of progress (Carver & Scheier, 1990). In short, rumination occurs when individuals are not making progress toward their higher-order goals. The goal-progress theory further assumes that the proximate underlying cause of rumination is the accessibility of goal-related information. Specifically, failure to attain a goal keeps information related to that goal highly accessible (Zeigarnik, 1938). When in this state, the information can be easily cued and is more likely to be used than equally relevant, but less accessible, information (e.g., Martin, Strack, & Stapel, 2001). As a result, otherwise innocuous stimuli might easily instigate rumination. This ruminative process explains why depressed patients are preoccupied with a sense of failure (unable to reduce symptoms and achieve higher-order goals) and in turn get caught in the vicious cycle of the depressive loop.

The left hemisphere follows well-practiced routines, whereas the right deviates from these routines (Burgess & Simpson, 1988). Rauch (1977) found that the left hemisphere tends to maintain pre-existing hypotheses even in the face of nonsupportive feedback, whereas the right hemisphere tends to switch even when its prior hypothesis was shown to be correct. These findings suggest that the left hemisphere tries to apply pre-existing structures, whereas the right hemisphere attempts to find alternatives to these structures. The tendency of the right hemisphere to provide alternative hypotheses fits the characterization of rumination as a search for alternative hypotheses (i.e., alternative paths to the goal). If the left hemisphere tends to operate from existing representations, then it may not be as useful as the right when individuals face a novel task. Here, the right hemisphere's ability to explore alternative strategies might facilitate the learning of new skills. Once the task is learned, however, the left hemisphere can take over again and guide behavior in accordance with its newly established representations. This analysis suggests a shift from right to left dominance as individuals move from learning a new task to performing a well-learned task (Gordon & Carmon, 1976; Goldberg & Costa, 1981). In ruminative terms, the right hemisphere is likely to become active in situations in which the established patterns are no longer applicable and individuals must think of alternatives. The right hemisphere is the locus of the Zeigarnik effect (Bowden & Beeman, 1998), that is, it maintains activation of information related to nonattained goals. Wegner, et al. (1987) have demonstrated the paradoxical or rebound effect of thought suppression. When ruminators "stop their active suppression, the heightened accessibility can lead the thought to return to mind at a level greater than if the individuals had not attempted to suppress the thought in the first place" (Martin, Shrira, & Startup, 2004, p. 163). According to the goal-progress view, the rebound reflects a failure to attain the higher-order goal of suppressing one's thoughts. Individuals who feel they are making little progress in their life in general may be more susceptible to the rebound effect. However, when individuals process positive information about themselves, the rebound effect is eliminated (Koole, et al., 1999). Evidence suggests (Don, 1977; Kuiken & Mathews, 1986–1987) that right hemisphere rumination can facilitate insight. Those experiencing positive moods stop worrying, whereas those experiencing negative moods continue to worry (Hirt, Levine, McDonald, Melton, & Martin, 1997). Rumination of catastrophic worries is a function of the perception of not achieving goal progress (Davey & Levy, 1998).

Moreover, negative mood makes high worriers continue worrying because they feel they have not made sufficient progress on their problem.

As discussed earlier, rumination has been found to be associated with depression (Morrow & Nolen-Hoeksema, 1990) and augmented pessimism (Lyubormirsky & Nole-Hoeksema, 1995). Right-hemisphere activation has been shown to be associated with greater negative affect (Merckelbach & Van Oppen, 1989), greater depression (Tomarken & Keener, 1998), more negative self-evaluation (Ahern, Herring, Tackenburg, & Schwartz, 1994), and greater pessimism (Drake & Ulrich, 1992). In addition, activation of the left hemisphere is associated with action, whereas activation of the right hemisphere is associated with a slowdown in action (Tucker & Williamson, 1984). So, when individuals are unable to rely upon established routines (left hemisphere) to proceed toward their goals, they search for alternatives. This search is associated with greater rumination, pessimism, sadness, depression, and negative self-evaluation, as well as a reduced tendency to act. From the evidence provided, it is clearly apparent that negative rumination plays a crucial part in both exacerbating and maintaining the depressive affect. Neuropsychophysiological studies provide a greater understanding of how different parts of the brain are involved in the ruminative process. Such understanding provides a rationale for the development of effective treatment intervention, for example, guiding the clinician to activate or deactivate certain parts of the brain via hypnotherapy to alleviate depressive symptoms and facilitate cognitive flexibility.

## Intensification of Negative Affect and Loss of Control

Dobson (1986) has reviewed the evidence for negative self-schemas in depression and has concluded that depressed patients view themselves as different from nondepressed patients. More centrally, the data show that depressed patients use cognitive style that differ from nondepressed persons to process information related to themselves and their experience. For example, Klinger et al. (1976), in a study of attention and recall, found subjects were (a) more likely to notice and attend to concern-related material than non–concern related material, and (b) more than twice as likely to recall concern-related material and to reflect on it in their spontaneous thoughts. In an unstructured situation, Klinger (1975) also noticed that severely depressed persons generated their own fear- and guilt-related cues, which led to a self-perpetuation and exacerbation of their depressive state. Moreover, rumination with such thematic contents (in daydreams, imagery, and stereotypic thinking) was converted into integrated components of their "inner reality" (repatterning and stabilization of baseline consciousness). However, the subjective sense of inner reality depends on the extent to which an experience is stabilized. As noted before, subjectivity or emotional involvement can lead to loss of control or dissociation (Bower, 1981). Horowitz (1972) has summarized the evidence for two types of subjective loss of control over the intensity of emotional imagery. In one type, the person experiences exceedingly intense images and is unable to avoid or dispel these experiences. In the other type of loss of control, the person is unable to form images that she subjectively wishes to have. Through such loss of control (dissociation), distortion, delusion, and errors can take place. As discussed earlier, rumination also contributes to loss of control via the rebound effect.

Imagery is also considered by CFMD to be an important aspect of cognition in determining, maintaining, and alleviating depression. Many writers (e.g., Ley & Freeman, 1984) claim that images have a greater capacity than language for attracting and retrieving emotionally laden associations. Individuals predisposed to depression tend to focus on negative thoughts and images. Schultz (1978, 1984, 2003), Starker and Singer (1975), and Traynor (1974) have provided evidence that, with increasing levels of depression, depressed patients tend to change the contents of their imagination to negative fantasies, and consequently they are unable to redirect their thinking and imagery from their current problems and negative life-concerns. Ley and Freeman (1984), from their review of the research on imagery and brain functions, concluded that "images can arouse strong emotions and vice versa is beyond question. One reason for this interdependence may be that the right cerebral hemisphere predominantly mediates both imagery and affect" (p. 54).

More recently, Nolen-Hoeksema (2004) has provided evidence that depressed patients have the tendency, or response style, to ruminate with their depressive symptoms and the consequences of their symptoms, resulting in the exacerbation and prolongation of the depressive symptoms. Such subjectivity or emotional involvement can lead to loss of control over the intensity of emotional imagery (Horowitz, 1972) or to the dissociation of affect (Bower, 1981). In other words, the circular feedback cycle between cognition and affect repeats itself almost like a computer caught in an infinite processing loop (Schultz, 1978) as the depression worsens, thus validating the depressive reality in the form of self-affirmations or posthypnotic suggestions. Such response style, according to Nolen-Hoeksema (2004), increases the likelihood of depressive symptoms becoming chronic, and of moderate symptoms evolving into episodes of major depression.

### Validation of Depressive Reality

Although we are capable of rational operations, most judgments are highly influenced by what is "available" (particularly vivid information) in current memory at the time (Kahneman, Slovic, & Tversky, 1982). Because depressed patients ruminate with negative self-schemas (Dobson, 1986), their judgments are likely to be biased, leading to the onset and maintenance of *syncretic cognition*. Syncretic cognition involves the fusion of various sources of information, such as visceral, postural, sensory, and mnemonic, to form an undifferentiated experiential matrix (Safer & Leventhal, 1977). Syncretic cognition, which is not unlike a hypnotic experience, can act as a powerful reinforcer in the validation of the depressive reality, both mentally and physically. It is worth mentioning that people don't normally validate their reality by how they think, but by their feelings.

To distinguish between the "nondepressed state" and the "depressive state" (conceptualized as a "dissociative state"),

Reality Perception = f( feelings )

and to further explore the cognitive processes involved in the phenomenology of depression, reference is made to the work of Hilgard (1977) and Tart (1975). As discussed in Chapter 3, Tart distinguishes among discrete states of consciousness (d-SOC), discrete altered state of consciousness (d-ASC), and baseline states of consciousness (b-SOC). A discrete altered state of consciousness (d-ASC) is different from baseline consciousness, consisting of a new system, generated from the restructuring of the cohesive self (consciousness or reality). In this sense, a hypnotic experience is a new experience (d-ASC) generated from the internal construction of existing cognitions (attitudes, feelings, motivations, and expectancies). This view can be easily extended to cognitive processing and organization in depression. In response to some negatively perceived external or internal stimuli, the existing cognitions (negative schemas) are repatterned (restructured or distorted), resulting in depressive affect (d-ASC). The intensity or severity of the affective symptoms will be determined by the progression and the degree of the repatterning of the existing negative schemas. As noted before (Chapter 3), new systems can take over from the executive ego (Hilgard, 1977). In the depressive state, automatic negative cognitions, depressive rumination, and the concomitant negative affect take over (split from b-SOC). Such an experience is not simply cognitive or affective, but "syncretic." The shift is away from acting on the world to experiencing it more directly. This involves becoming dissociated from ordinary concepts or categories of experience to direct mirroring of experience. In other words, the depressive state represents experiences without language or logical categories, and they occur effortlessly or spontaneously in response to internal and/or external cues. This process becomes the depressive reality created by repetitive cognitive distortions and depressive rumination. A nondepressive state, on the other hand, is composed of conceptual, analytical, and logical representations of the world, which act as a model of real reality.

However, we do not operate directly on the world; instead, we create a map or a model (schema), which we use to guide our experience and behaviors. Therefore, to a large extent, this model determines how we will perceive the world and what our attitudes, values, and motivations will be. Hypnotic strategies attempt to alter the way we represent our experience. During the hypnotic experience, baseline reality is distorted and modified, and a new system (d-ASC), with unique properties, is generated. This new system is stabilized (becomes a discrete reality) by syncretic cognition and the presence of associated internal and external feedback systems that occurred during the construction process (structuring of the hypnotic experience). Similarly, cognitive distortions may lead to a depressogenic schema, which can become stabilized by the depressive reality (depressive affect and associated physiological and psychological symptoms) and external factors such as adverse life events, loss of control over images, low threshold of information processing, and emotional responding. In other words, depression is reconstructed reality, based on negative self-schemas, validated by negative syncretic cognitions, and often resulting from adverse life events.

**Conscious and Unconscious Information Processing**

CFMD also attaches importance to nonconscious information processing. Judgments and emotions can be influenced by nonconscious cognitive processes (e.g., Kihlstrom, 1999; LeDoux, 2000; Williams, Watts, MacLeod, & Mathews, 1997). Shevrin and Dickman (1980), after reviewing the research evidence for nonconscious processes, concluded that no psychological model of human experience could ignore the concept of unconscious psychological processes. Work on selective attention (Posner, 1973; Sternberg, 1975) and subliminal perception (Shevrin, 1978) suggests that conscious psychological processes can be influenced by the initial phase of cognitive activity that occurs outside of awareness. These studies provide evidence that nonconscious processes may determine to a great extent what enters conscious awareness. Therefore, when a person is presented with a stimulus or situation, the person may be upset without knowing why (because nonconscious thinking or evaluation may be involved). Williams, et al. (1988), from their review of experimental evidence of nonconscious cognitive processes, conclude that some nonconscious psychological processes may have laws of organization different from conscious processes. More recent work in cognitive psychology proposes that a structural dissociation exists between conscious and unconscious processes (e.g., Reber, 1993; Seger, 1992). This proposition is succinctly summarized by David and Szentagotai (2006, pp. 288–289):

Some aspects of information processing (including both perceptual and semantic processing), by their characteristics, cannot be made conscious. They are represented in our memory in a format (e.g., nonverbal associations) that is not consciously accessible (Schacter & Tulving, 1994). These non-declarative/implicit memory processes (structurally separated from consciousness and not consciously accessible) exert a major impact on interpersonal experience, emotions, cognitions, and behavior, independent of beliefs, and they need to be analyzed on their own terms. They should not be mistakenly viewed as a form of repressed memory or only as an automatization (functionally separated from consciousness and consciously accessible) of explicit memory processes (e.g., beliefs) (Tobias, Kihlstrom, & Schacter, 1992). Some "Cs" (e.g., feelings) are not mediated by beliefs at all, but instead, by unconscious information processing, which is structurally separated from consciousness (e.g., nonverbal associations) (LeDoux, 2000).

These recent developments from cognitive psychology have widened our understanding, assessment, and treatment of the depressive state. These understandings encouraged me to combine hypnosis with CBT. CBT, which relies on recognition and alteration of conscious cognitions, may be ineffective here. Hypnotherapy provides several strategies for accessing and restructuring nonconscious information. The integration of conscious and nonconscious information processing within the CFMD has expanded the psychotherapeutic intervention for depression. Several techniques for dealing with nonconscious cognitive influence in depression are described in Chapter 10.

### The Role of Undesirable Life Events

So far, the discussion has centered on information processing in depression, rumination, and hypnosis, with no mention made of trigger factors (internal or external), the role of biological variables, or the influence of early experience that contributes to the genesis, onset, and maintenance of clinical depression. The important question still remains: What are the factors that contribute to the construction and consolidation of the depressive reality? Paykel, Myers, Dienelt, Klerman, Lindenthal, and Pepper (1969) and Schultz (1978) have noted more frequent undesirable life events (e.g., changes in sleep pattern, personal injury or illness, financial problems, troubles with spouse, sexual problems, etc.) among depressed patients as compared with the general population. Beck (1967) and Schultz (1978) argue that such undesirable life-event factors may contribute to the depressive cycle in depressed patients. Schultz (1978) further argues that once undesirable life events are introduced into the depressive loop process, the incidence of negative events is increased. Because of their underlying negative self-schemas (cognitive triad), depressed patients tend to become inactive and "careless" in the face of undesirable life events, thus scaffolding more negative events. For example, a construction worker on long-term disability for depression neglected to pay for two speeding tickets (booked for overspeeding on two occasions) and was summoned to appear in court. This incident prolonged his depressive state. Moreover, the depressed patient's ruminations on the belief that negative life events will always haunt them, and that they will not be able to cope with them in the future, leads to catastrophic reactions to any undesirable life events (far beyond what they would have been if the person was not depressed).

Studies have been conducted to examine the association between depressive rumination and undesirable life events. The *response styles theory* of depression discussed earlier (under Depressive Rumination) has been extended to encompass the cognitive and the hopelessness theories of depression. In this extension theory, Alloy and his colleagues (Alloy, Abramson, Hogan, Whitehouse, Rose, Robinson, Kim, & Lapkin, 2000; Robinson & Alloy, 2003) developed the concept of *stress-reactive rumination* to refer to the tendency to ruminate on negative inferences following stressful life events. Within this conceptualization, stress-reactive rumination occurs prior to the onset of depressed mood, whereas *emotion-focused rumination*, as proposed by Nolen-Hoeksema (1991), occurs in response to depressed mood. Alloy and Abramson (1999) presented data from the Temple-Wisconsin Cognitive Vulnerability to Depression Project (see Chapter 2) to demonstrate that stress-reactive rumination plays a crucial role in the etiology of depression. They found the interaction between negative cognitive styles and stress-reactive rumination predicted the retrospective lifetime rate of major depressive episodes as well as hopelessness depressive episodes. In a subsequent study (Robinson & Alloy, 2003), they found the same interaction to predict prospective onset, number, and duration of major depressive and hopelessness depressive episodes.

**Symbolic Transformation**

The works of Brown and Harris (1978) and Schultz (1978) have shown little correlation between undesirable life events and severity of depression. Klinger (1975) points out that the "symbolic transformation" of these events is the critical factor. He suggests undesirable life events may serve as cues to past traumatic experiences.

**Anchoring, Kindling, Biogenic Changes, and Development of Depressive Pathways**

Depressed patients gradually not only become more sensitive to stimuli resembling past traumatic life events, but their reactions may also generalize to innocuous events or situations. Such selective attending or "anchoring" may explain the low threshold of information processing to emotional stimuli in depressed patients. Through repeated and automatic anchoring, biogenic changes may occur. Schwartz (1977, 1984; Schwartz, Fair, Salt, Mandel, & Klerman, 1976) has provided evidence for the development of certain neurological pathways due to conscious cognitive focusing. Since depressed patients tend to automatically focus on negative cognitions, and are hypervalent to negative stimuli because of their low threshold of emotional information processing, they can easily develop "depressive pathways." It is also possible for some individuals who are predisposed to depression to already possess a depressive pathway as a result of their developmental history. Psychiatric disorders are often associated with stressful early life experiences and anomalous developmental processes (Guidano, 1987). Such experiences and patterns of development can have differing effects on each part of the brain (Wexler, 1980), especially as different parts of the brain contain different levels of bioamines (Oke, Keller, Mefford, & Adams, 1978). So it is not only existent or latent depressive pathways that predispose an individual to depression, but the symbolic transformation of past emotional traumas also can predispose an individual to depression. Individuals with anomalous developmental history (Guidano, 1987) and those who are biologically vulnerable (Oke, et al., 1978) or genetically predisposed to depression will be more prone to develop these depressive pathways. The *kindling hypothesis* (Post, 1992) provides some evidence for the development of increasing sensitization in individuals prone to depression.

Neurons that are repeatedly subjected to convulsions or electrical stimuli show a process of *kindling* (Cleare, 2004), whereby the convulsive threshold is gradually lowered, and the neurons eventually fire autonomously. Post (1992) suggested that kindling may underlie the tendency for some depressed patients to suffer increasingly severe or refractory episodes of depression, or to require fewer provoking life events with passing time. Segal, Williams, and Teasdale (1996) posited that an elaborate network of depression-related material becomes activated when a person is depressed. This activation promotes negative processing of stimuli, and it sets in motion a vicious cycle, making it harder to activate areas that could disconfirm negative thoughts, and thereby maintaining a negative affect. Recurrence of depression is therefore conceptualized as a lowered activational threshold for depressogenic structures or schemas in the presence of dysphoric affect. Those with early negative life experiences and an accompanying experience of sadness might also experience concomitant activation of negative thoughts. Segal, et al. (1996) proposed that increased activation increases accessibility to such sad-related thoughts as worthlessness and hopelessness so that patients begin to associate sadness with adversity. Gradually, depressogenic schemas can become strongly associated and more generalized so that, over time, many more contexts can activate the depressed affect and depressive thinking.

Strong support for the kindling hypothesis was provided by Kendler, Thornton, and Gardner (2000), who followed over 2,000 community-based female twin pairs over 9 years, measuring depression and life-event severity during this period. They found a clear tendency for each episode of depression to be followed by an increased subsequent risk of a further episode of depression less strongly related to preceding life stress. Post (1992) suggested that the increased vulnerability for recurrence of depression occurs at the neuronal level, and each episode leaves a neurobiological trace. More recently, Monroe and Harkness (2005) have provided an integrative model to explain the role of kindling in the recurrence of depression in the context of life stress. In Part III, several techniques are described to modulate the kindling effect.

**Hopelessness**

Our present mood state and self-esteem are not only influenced by our past and present experiences, but they also determine our future responses and expectations. Because their cognitive distortions become hypervalent during depression, depressed patients tend to think more negatively (Beck, et al., 1979) and hence they perceive the future as a continuous pattern of failure, relentless hardship, and inability to cope. This anticipation of failure (syncretic cognition associated with negative thoughts and images) creates a projected poor self-image in the future, which in terms of NSH, promotes a dissociated depressive reality. This negative syncretic cognition coupled with the hypervalent depressive schemas creates a sense of helplessness and hopelessness. These feelings are further exacerbated if the individual lacks social and problem-solving skills (Youngren & Lewinshon, 1980) and/or is surrounded by adverse environmental factors (poor housing, unemployment, etc.) (Paykel, et al., 1969), and/or lacks social support (Brown & Harris, 1978). These factors help to reinforce and consolidate/stabilize the negative schemas (negative affirmations/posthypnotic suggestions), and thus a sense of despair and hopelessness sets in. At this point, depressed patients are most vulnerable to suicide. Moreover, the distress, despair, sense of hopelessness, and lack of motivation may increase the negative affect and the vegetative symptoms, thus allowing the depressive loop to continue to reverberate.

**SUMMARY**

CFMD is not another theory of depression, but an extension of Beck's cognitive theory of depression. The model emphasizes functional autonomy and circular causality, so that factors such as cognitive distortions, negative ruminations, distressed relationships, adverse life events, and neurochemical changes are seen as both symptoms and causes at the same time. Any of the 12 components in the loop can trigger depression, and the interrelationship among the components allows the depressive loop to continue to reverberate. The purpose of therapy is to break the depressive loop and teach patients a variety of skills to counter the factors that lead to the reverberation of the depressive cycle. The conceptualization of nonendogenous unipolar depression as a form of dissociation is innovative and provocative, and it is likely to generate debate. Furthermore, the psychobiological nature of depression is emphasized by incorporating undesirable life events, genetic predisposition, depressive pathways and cerebral laterality into the model. The model also highlights the importance of both conscious and nonconscious cognitive processes. Empirical investigation of the model is likely to refine the CDMD and advance our understanding of the construction of the depressive reality. The next chapter discusses the clinical implications of the model.

## REFERENCES

Ahern, G.L., Herring, A.M., Tackenburg, J.N., & Schwartz, G.E. (1994). Affective self-report during the intracarotid test. *Journal of Clinical and Experimental Neuropsychology*, 16, 372–376.

Akiskal, H.S., & McKinney, W.I. (1975). Overview of recent research in depression: Integration of ten conceptual models into a comprehensive clinical frame. *Archives of General Psychiatry*, 32, 285–305.

Alladin, A. (1989). Cognitive hypnotherapy for depression. In D. Waxman, D. Pederson, I. Wilkie, & P. Mellett (Eds.), *Hypnosis: The 4th European Congress at Oxford* (pp. 175–182). London: Whurr Publishers.

Alladin, A. (1992). Depression as a dissociative state. *Hypnos: Swedish Journal of Hypnosis in Psychotherapy and Psychosomatic Medicine*, 19, 243–253.

Alladin, A. (1994). Cognitive hypnotherapy with depression. *Journal of Cognitive Psychotherapy: An International Quarterly*, 8(4), 275–288.

Alladin, A. (2005). *Cognitive hypnotherapy for depression: An empirical investigation*. Paper presented at the American Psychological Association Annual Convention, Washington, DC, August 2005.

Alladin, A. (2006). Cognitive hypnotherapy for treating depression. In R. Chapman (Ed.), *The clinical use of hypnosis with cognitive behavior therapy: A practitioner's casebook* (pp. 139–187). New York: Springer Publishing Company.

Alladin, A. (2006a). Experiential cognitive hypnotherapy: Strategies for relapse prevention in depression. In M. Yapko (Ed.), *Hypnosis and treating depression: Advances in clinical practice* (pp. 281–313). New York: Routledge, Taylor & Francis Group.

Alladin, A., & Alibhai, A. (2007). Cognitive hypnotherapy therapy for depression: An empirical investigation. *International Journal of Clinical and Experimental Hypnosis*, in press.

Alladin, A., & Heap, M. (1991). Hypnosis and depression. In M. Heap & W. Dryden (Eds.), *Hypnotherapy: A handbook* (pp. 49–67). Milton Keynes: Open University Press.

Alloy, L.B., & Abramson, L.Y. (1999). The Temple-Wisconsin Cognitive Vulnerability to Depression (CVD) project: Conceptual background, design and methods. *Journal of Cognitive Psychotherapy: An International Quarterly*, 13, 227–262.

Alloy, L.B., Abramson, L.Y., Hogan, M.E., Whitehouse, W.G., Rose, D.T., Robinson, M.S., Kim, R.S., & Lapkin, J.B. (2000). The Temple-Wisconsin Cognitive Vulnerability to Depression (CVD) Project: Lifetime history of Axis I psychopathology in individuals at high and low cognitive risk for depression. *Journal of Abnormal Psychology*, 109, 403–418.

Araoz, D.L. (1981). Negative self-hypnosis. *Journal of Contemporary Psychotherapy*, 12, 45–52.

Araoz, D.L. (1985). *The new hypnosis*. New York: Brunner-Mazel.

Beck, A.T. (1967). *Depression: Clinical, experimental and theoretical aspects*. New York: Hoeber.

Beck, A.T., Rush, A.J., Shaw, B.F., & Emery, G. (1979). *Cognitive therapy of depression*. New York: Guilford Press.

Bowden, E.M., & Beeman, M.J. (1998). Getting the right idea: Semantic activation in the right hemisphere may help solve insight problems. *Psychological Science*, 9, 435–440.

Bower, G. (1981). Mood and memory. *American Psychologist*, 36, 129–148.

Brown, G.W., & Harris, T. (1978). *Social origins of depression*. New York: The Free Press.

Burgess, C., & Simpson, G.B. (1988). Cerebral hemispheric mechanisms in the retrieval of ambiguous word meanings. *Brain and Language*, 33, 86–103.

Burrows, G.D., & Broughton, S.G. (2001). Hypnosis and depression. In G.D. Burrows, R.O. Stanley, & P.B. Bloom (Eds.), *International handbook of clinical hypnosis* (pp. 129–142). New York: Wiley.

Calkins, S.D., Fox, N.A., & Marshall, T.R. (1996). Behavioral and physiological antecedents of inhibited and uninhibited behavior. *Child Development*, 67, 523–540.

Carver, C.S., & Scheier, M.F. (1990). Origins and functions of positive and negative affect: A control-process view. *Psychological Review*, 97, 19–35.

Chambless, D.L. and Hollon, S.D. (1998). Defining empirically-supported therapies. *Journal of Consulting and Clinical Psychology*, 66, 7–18.

Cleare, A.J. (2004). Biological models of unipolar depression. In M. Power (Ed.), *Mood disorders: A handbook of science and practice* (pp. 29–46). Chichester: John Wiley & Sons, Ltd.

Crawford, H., & Gruzelier, J. (1992). A midstream of the neuropsychophysiology of hypnosis: Recent research and future directions. In E. Fromm & M. Nash (Eds.), *Contemporary hypnosis research* (pp. 227–266). New York: Guildford.

Davey, G.C.L., & Levy, S. (1998). Catastrophic worrying: Personal inadequacy and a perseverative iterative style as features of the catastrophizing process. *Journal of Abnormal Psychology*, 107, 576–586.

David, D., & Szentagotai, A. (2006). Cognitions in cognitive-behavioral psychotherapies; toward an integrative model. *Clinical Psychology Review*, 26, 284–298.

Davidson, R.J., Pizzagalli, D, & Nitschke, J.B. (2002). The representation and regulation of emotion in depression: Perspectives from affective neuroscience. In I.H. Gotlib & C.L. Hammen (Eds.), *Handbook of depression* (pp. 219–244). New York: The Guilford Press.

De Pascalis, V. (1999). Psychophysiological correlates of hypnosis and hypnotic susceptibility.

Dobson, K.S. (1986). The self-schema in depression. In L.M. Hartmen & K.R. Blankstein (Eds.), *Perception of self in emotional disorder and psychotherapy* (pp. 187–217). New York: Plenum Press.

Don, N.S. (1977). The transformation of conscious experience and its EEG correlates. *Journal of Altered States of Consciousness, 3*, 147–168.

Drake, R.A., & Ulrich, G. (1992). Line bisecting as a predictor of personal optimism and desirability of risky behaviors. *Acta Psychologica, 79*, 219–226.

Easterbrook, J.A. (1959). The effect of emotion on cue utilization and the organization of behavior. *Psychological Review, 56*, 183–201.

Ebert, D., Feistel, H., Kaschka, W., Barocka, A., & Pirner, A. (1994). Single photon emission computerized tomography assessment of cerebral dopamine D2 receptor blockade in depression before and after sleep deprivation—Preliminary results. *Biological Psychiatry, 35*, 880–885.

Ekman, P., Davidson, R.J., & Friesen, W.V. (1990). The Duchenne smile: Emotional expression and brain physiology II. *Journal of Personality and Social Psychology, 58*, 342–353.

Fry, P.S. (1977). Success, failure, and resistance to temptation. *Developmental Psychology, 13*, 519–520.

Gilbert, P. (2004). Depression: A biopsychosocial, integrative, and evolutionary approach. In M. Power (Ed.), *Mood disorders: A handbook of science and practice* (pp. 99–142). Chichester: John Wiley & Sons, Ltd.

Goldberg, E., & Costa, L.D. (1981). Hemisphere differences in the acquisition and use of descriptive systems. *Brain and Language, 14*, 144–173.

Golden, W.L., Dowd, E.T., & Friedberg, F. (1987). *Hypnotherapy: A modern approach.* New York: Pergamon Press.

Gordon, H.W., & Carmon, A. (1976). Transfer of dominance in speed of verbal response to visually presented stimuli from right to left hemisphere. *Perceptual and Motor Skills, 42*, 1091–1100.

Graham, K.R. (1977). Perceptual processes and hypnosis: Support for a cognitive-state theory based on laterality. In W.E. Edmonston, Jr. (Ed.), Conceptual and investigative approaches to hypnosis and hypnotic phenomena. *Annals of New York Academy of Sciences, 296*, 274–283.

Gruzelier, J. (2000). Redefining hypnosis: Theory, methods and integration. *Contemporary Hypnosis, 17*, 51–70.

Guidano, V.F. (1987). *Complexity of the self: A developmental approach to psychopathology and therapy.* New York: Guilford Press.

Haaga, D.A.F., Dyck, M.J., & Ernst, D. (1991). Empirical status of cognitive therapy of depression. *Psychological Bulletin, 110*, 215–236.

Haas, G.L., & Fitzgibbon, M.L. (1989). In J.J. Mann (Ed.), *Models of depressive disorders* (pp. 9–43). New York: Plenum Press.

Hartland, J. (1971). *Medical and dental hypnosis and its clinical applications* (2nd ed.). London: Bailliere Tindall.

Henriques, J.B., & Davidson, R.J. (1990). Regional brain electrical asymmetries discriminate between previously depressed subjects and healthy controls. *Journal of Abnormal Psychology*, 99, 22–31.

Hilgard, E.R. (1977). *Divided consciousness: Multiple controls in human thought and action*. New York: John Wiley & Sons.

Hirt, E.R., Levine, G.M., McDonald, H.E., Melton, R.J., & Martin, L.L. (1997). The role of mood in quantitative and qualitative aspects of performance: Single or multiple mechanisms? *Journal of Experimental Social Psychology*, 33, 602–629.

Horowitz, M.J. (1972). Image formation: Clinical observation and a cognitive model. In P.W. Sheehan (Ed.), *The function and nature of imagery* (pp. 282–309). New York: Academic Press.

*International Journal of Clinical and Experimental Hypnosis*, 47, 117–143.

Jaynes, J. (1976). *The origin of consciousness in the breakdown of the bicameral mind*. Boston: Houghton Mifflin Co.

Kahneman, D., Slovic, P., & Tversky, A. (1882). *Judgment under uncertainty: Heuristics and biases*. Cambridge: Cambridge University Press.

Kendler, K.S., Thornton, L.M., & Gardner, C.O. (2000). Genetic risk, number of previous depressive episodes, and stressful life events in predicting onset of major depression. *American Journal of Psychiatry*, 158, 582–586.

Kihlstrom, J.F. (1999). Conscious versus unconscious cognition. In R.J. Sternberg (Ed.), *The concept of cognition* (pp. 173–204). Cambridge: MIT Press.

Kirsch, I., Montgomery, G., & Sapirstein, G. (1995). Hypnosis as an adjunct to cognitive-behavioral psychotherapy: A meta-analysis. *Journal of Consulting and Clinical Psychology*, 63, 214–220.

Klinger, E. (1975). The nature of fantasy and its clinical uses. In J.L. Klinger (Chair), *Imagery approaches to psychotherapy*. Symposium presented at the Meeting of the American Psychological Association, Chicago.

Klinger, E., Barta, S.G., Mahoney, T.W., et al. (1976). Motivation, mood, and mental events: Patterns and implications for adaptive processes. In G. Serban (Ed.), *Psychopathology of human adaptation* (pp. 95–112). New York: Plenum.

Koole, S.L., Smeets, K., van Knippenberg, A., & Dijksterhuis, A. (1999). The cessation of rumination through self-affirmation. *Journal of Personality and Social Psychology*, 77, 111–125.

Kuiken, D., & Mathews, J. (1986–1987). EEG and facial EMG changes during self-reflection with affective imagery. *Imagination, Cognition, and Personality*, 6, 55–66.

LeDoux, J.E. (2000). Emotion circuits in the brain. *Annual Review of Neuroscience*, 23, 155–184.

Ley, R.G., & Freeman, R.J. (1984). Imagery, cerebral laterality, and the healing process. In A.A. Sheikh (Ed.), *Imagination and healing* (pp. 51–68). New York: Baywood.

Lyubormirsky, S., & Nolen-Hoeksema, S. (1995). Self-perpetuating properties of dysphoric rumination. *Journal of Personality and Social Psychology*, 65, 339–349.

Lyubomirsky, S., & Tkach, C. (2004). The consequences of dysphoric rumination. In C. Papageorgiou & A. Wells (Eds.), *Depressive rumination: Nature theory and treatment* (pp. 21–41). Chichester: John Wiley & Sons, Ltd.

Martin, L.L., Shrira, I., & Startup, H.M. (2004). Rumination as a function of goal progress, stop rules, and cerebral lateralization. In C. Papageorgiou & A. Wells (Eds.), *Depressive rumination: Nature theory and treatment* (pp. 153–175). Chichester: John Wiley & Sons, Ltd.

Martin, L.L., Strack, F., & Stapel, D.A. (2001). How the mind moves: Knowledge accessibility and the fine-tuning of the cognitive system. In A. Tesser & N. Schwarz (Eds.), Blackwell International *Handbook of Social Psychology: Intra-individual Processes* (Vol. 1, pp. 236–256). London: Blackwell.

Mayberg, H.S. (2006). Brain imaging. In D.J. Stein, D.J. Kupfer, & A.F. Schatzberg (Eds.), *Textbook of mood disorders* (pp. 219–234). Washington, DC: American Psychiatric Publishing, Inc.

Merckelbach, H., & Van Oppen, P. (1989). Effects of gaze manipulation on subjective evaluation of neutral and phobia-relevant stimuli: A comment on Drake's (1987) "Effects of gaze manipulation on aesthetic judgments: Hemispheric priming of affect." *Acta Psychologica*, 70, 147–151.

Monroe, S.M., & Harkness, K.L. (2005). Life stress, the "kindling" hypothesis, and the recurrence of depression: Considerations from life stress perspectives. *Psychological Review*, 112, 417–445.

Morrow, J., & Nolen-Hoeksema, S. (1990). Effects of responses to depression on the remediation of depressive affect. *Journal of Personality and Social Psychology*, 58, 519–527.

Neisser, U. (1967). *Cognitive Psychology*. New York: Appleton-Century-Croft.

Nemeroff, C.B. (2000). An ever-increasing pharmacopoeia for the management of patients with bipolar disorder. *Journal of Clinical Psychiatry*, 65(Suppl. 1), 18–28.

Nolen-Hoeksema, S. (1991). Responses to depression and their effects on the duration of depressive episodes. *Journal of Abnormal Psychology*, 100, 569–582.

Nolen-Hoeksema, S. (2000). The role of rumination in depressive disorders and mixed anxiety/depressive symptoms. *Journal of Abnormal Psychology*, 109, 504–511.

Nolen-Hoeksema, S. (2004). *Abnormal Psychology* (3rd ed.). New York: McGraw-Hill.

Oke, A., Keller, R., Mefford, I., & Adams, R.N. (1978). Lateralization of norepinephrine in human thalamus. *Science*, 200, 1411–1433.

Papageorgiou, C., & Wells, A. (1999). Process and metacognitive dimensions of depressive and anxious thoughts and relationships with emotional intensity. *Clinical Psychology and Psychotherapy*, 6, 156–162.

Papageorgiou, C., & Wells, A. (2004). Nature, functions, and beliefs about depressive rumination. In C. Papageorgiou & A. Wells (Eds.), *Depressive rumination: Nature theory and treatment* (pp. 3–20). Chichester: John Wiley & Sons, Ltd.

Paykel, E.S., Meyers, J.K., Dienett, M.N., Klerman, G.L., Linderthal, J.J., & Pepper, M.P. (1969). Life events and depression: A controlled study. *Archives of General Psychiatry*, 21, 753–760.

Posner, M.I. (1973). *Cognition: An introduction*. Glenview, IL: Scott, Foresman.

Post, M.I. (1992). Transduction of psychosocial stress into the neurobiology of recurrent affective disorder. *American Journal of Psychiatry*, 149, 999–1010.

Rauch, R. (1977). Cognitive strategies in patients with unilateral temporal lobe excisions. *Neuropsychologica*, 15, 385–395.

Reber, A.S. (1993). *Implicit learning and tacit knowledge: An essay in the cognitive unconscious*. Oxford: Oxford University Press.

Rippere, V. (1977). "What's the thing to do when you're depressed?"— A pilot study. *Behavior Research and Therapy*, 15, 185–191.

Robinson, S.M., & Alloy, L.B. (2003). Negative cognitive styles and stress-reactive rumination interact to predict depression: A prospective study. *Cognitive Therapy and Research*, 27, 275–291.

Safer, M.A., & Leventhal, H. (1977). Ear differences in evaluating emotional tone of voice and verbal content. *Journal of Experimental Psychology: Human Perception and Performance*, 3, 75–82.

Schoenberger, N.E. (2000). Research on hypnosis as an adjunct to cognitive-behavioral psychotherapy. *International Journal of Clinical and Experimental Hypnosis*, 48, 154–169.

Schultz, K.D. (1978). Imagery and the control of depression. In J.L. Singer & K.S. Pope (Eds.), *The power of human imagination: New methods in psychotherapy* (pp. 281–307). New York: Plenum Press.

Schultz, K.D. (1984). The use of imagery in alleviating depression. In A.A. Sheik (Ed.), *Imagination and healing* (pp. 129–158). New York: Baywood.

Schultz, K.D. (2003). The use of imagery in alleviating depression. In A.A. Sheikh (Ed.), *Healing images: The role of imagination in health* (pp. 343–380). New York: Baywood.

Schwartz, G. (1977). Psychosomatic disorders in biofeedback: A psychological model of disregulation. In J.D. Maser & M.E.P. Seligman (Eds.), *Psychopathology: Experimental models* (pp. 270–307). San Francisco: W.H. Freeman.

Schwartz, G. (1984). Psychophysiology of imagery and healing: A systems perspective. In A.A. Sheik (Ed.), *Imagination and healing* (pp. 35–50). New York: Baywood.

Schwartz, G., Fair, P.L., Salt, P., Mandel, M.R., & Klerman, G.L. (1976). Facial muscle patterning in affective imagery in depressed and non-depressed subjects. *Science*, 192, 489–491.

Segal, Z.V., Williams, J.M., Teasdale, J., & Gemar, M. (1996). A cognitive science perspective on kindling and episode sensitization in recurrent affective disorder. *Psychological Medicine*, 26, 371–380.

Seger, C.A. (1992). *Implicit learning*. UCLA Cognitive Science Research Program Technical Report #UCLA-CSRP-92-3.

Sheehan, P.W. (1992). The phenomenology of hypnosis and experiential analysis technique. In E. Fromm & M.R. Nash (Eds.), *Contemporary Hypnosis Research* (pp. 364–389). New York: Guilford Press.

Shevrin, H. (1978). Evoked potential evidence for unconscious mental process: A review of the literature. In A.S. Prangishvili, A.E. Sherozia, & F.V. Bassin (Eds.), *The unconscious: Nature, functions, methods of study*. Tbilisi, USSR, Metsnierba.

Shevrin, H., & Dickman, S. (1980). The psychologically unconscious American. *American Psychologist*, 5, 421.

Spiegel, H., & Spiegel, D. (2004). *Trance and treatment: Clinical uses of hypnosis* (2nd ed.). Washington, DC: American Psychiatric Publishing, Inc.

Starker, S., & Singer, J.L. (1975). Daydreaming patterns of self-awareness in psychiatric patients. *Journal of Nervous and Mental Disease*, 163, 313–317.

Sternberg, S. (1975). Memory scanning: New findings and current controversies. *Quarterly Journal of Experimental Psychology*, 27, 1.

Tart, C. (1975). *States of consciousness*. New York: Dutton.

Tomarken, A.J., & Keener, A.D. (1998). Frontal brain asymmetry and depression: A self-regulatory perspective. *Cognition and Emotion*, 12, 387–420.

Tosi, D. J., & Baisden, B.S. (1984). Cognitive-experiential therapy and hypnosis. In W.C. Wester & A.H. Smith (Eds.), *Clinical hypnosis: A multidisciplinary approach* (pp. 155–178). Philadelphia: J.B. Lippincott Co.

Traynor, J.D. (1974). *Patterns of daydreaming and their relationship to depressive affect*. Unpublished masters thesis. Miami University, Oxford, Ohio.

Tucker, D.M., & Williamson, P.A. (1984). Asymmetric neural control systems in human self-regulation. *Psychological Review*, 91, 185–215.

Wegner, D.M., Schneider, D.J., Carter, S.R., & White, T.L. (1987). Paradoxical effects of thought suppression. *Journal of Personality and Social Psychology*, 53, 5–13.

Williams, J.M.G., Watts, F.N., MacLeod, C., & Mathews, A. (1997). *Cognitive psychology and emotional disorders*. Chichester: John Wiley & Sons, Ltd.

Yapko, M.D. (1992). *Hypnosis and the treatment of depressions: Strategies for change*. New York: Brunner-Mazel.

Yapko, M.D. (2001). *Treating depression with hypnosis: Integrating cognitive-behavioral and strategic approaches*. Philadelphia: Brunner-Rutledge.

Yapko, M.D. (2003). *Trancework: An introduction to the practice of clinical hypnosis* (3rd ed.). New York: Brunner-Routledge.

Youngren, M.A., & Lewinshon, P.M. (1980). The functional relation between depression and problematic interpersonal behavior. *Journal of Abnormal Psychology*, 89, 333–341.

Zeigarnik, B. (1938). On finished and unfinished tasks. In W.D. Ellis (Ed.), *A source book of gestalt psychology* (pp. 300–314). New York: Harcourt, Brace, & World.

# 5

# Clinical Implications and Empirical Evidence

The *circular feedback model of depression* (CFMD) takes a multidimensional view of depression. The 12 factors forming the depressive loop are all interrelated, forming a constellation of emotional, cognitive, behavioral, physiological, and nonconscious processes. Focusing on any of the factors allows the patient and the therapist a point of entry into the depressive loop. Which point of entry is selected is determined by the case formulation. Once the patient and the therapist gain access into this set of relationships, they can deploy various techniques as tools to unravel and reorganize this interrelated set. Part III of the book describes various empirical and principle-based intervention strategies. Any of the factors identified by the case formulation can be used as a target for intervention, which can influence simultaneously other processes because of their interrelated nature (Simons, Garfield, & Murphy, 1984). Because depression is a complex disorder involving multiple risk factors and is often comorbid with other conditions, it is unlikely that a single causative factor, either biological or psychological, will be found. Similarly any single intervention is unlikely to provide long-term benefits, although focusing on any of the set of factors may be sufficient to bring on symptomatic relief. The therapist is encouraged to use multiple interventions. Williams (1992), in his comprehensive review of the psychotherapies for depression, concluded that the more techniques that are used, the more effective is the treatment, especially in the prevention of future relapses (Kovacs, et al., 1981). Many studies have demonstrated the superiority of combined treatments (Blackburn, et al., 1981; Taylor & Marshall, 1977; Weissman, et al., 1979, 1981) over single modality therapies. The poorest outcomes tend to result from the strategy that uses the smallest number of techniques. This suggests that the more techniques over which a therapist is allowed to range, the more likely it is that a combination will be found that is maximally suitable for the particular characteristics of her patients.

*Cognitive hypnotherapy* (CH) provides this multifactorial treatment approach to depression, and allows the therapist to easily combine the most appropriate strategies to suit a particular patient. Although this treatment approach primarily combines cognitive therapy with hypnotherapeutic techniques, it also makes use of behavioral, affective, psychodynamic, and imagery techniques. The therapist should refrain, however, from utilizing random techniques in a shotgun fashion. Instead, the techniques chosen should match the patient's needs, as determined by the case formulation, and use evidence-based interventions to strengthen

**Table 5.1.   Stages of cognitive hypnotherapy
for depression**

- First Aid for Depression
- Cognitive Therapy
- Hypnotherapy
- Cognitive Hypnotherapy
- Positive Mood Induction
- Active-Interactive Training
- Physical Exercises and Behavioral Assignments
- Social Skills/Assertive Training
- Reality and Mindfulness Training
- Relapse Prevention

the empirical foundation of CH as a treatment for depression. The clinician can become more effective at reducing a patient's distress when treatment selection is based on a thorough understanding of the patient's reality, rather than an imposition of the therapist's reality (theoretical orientation) on the patient. Because research indicates that depressive pathways can be developed, then, conversely, it should be possible to stimulate and develop antidepressive pathways. Later in this chapter, several hypnotic and imagery techniques are described for developing such pathways.

CH normally consists of 16 weekly sessions (see Alladin, 2006), which can be expanded or modified according to patient's clinical needs, areas of concern, and presenting symptoms. The stages of CH are listed in Table 5.1, and they are described in detail in Chapters 7 to 15. The sequence of treatment stages can be altered to suit the clinical needs of the individual patient.

**EFFECTIVENESS OF COGNITIVE HYPNOTHERAPY**

The effectiveness of CH with depression has been empirically validated. We (Alladin, 2005; Alladin & Alibhai, 2007) conducted a randomized study to compare the effects of CH with a well-established treatment, cognitive behavioral therapy (CBT), with a sample of chronically depressed patients. The study met all APA Task Force (Chambless & Hollon, 1998) criteria for probably efficacious treatment. Ninety-eight chronic outpatient depressed patients were randomly assigned to either CH or CBT. Eighty-four patients completed the 16-week outpatient treatment, and were followed-up at 6 and 12 months. CBT was based on the manual produced by Beck, et al. (1979), and the CH was based on a paper by the author (Alladin, 1994) that was extended into a treatment manual. In addition to CBT, the CH group had hypnotherapy consisting of (a) counting, using the relaxation method of hypnotic induction and deepening of trance (adapted from Gibbons, 1979), (b) ego-strengthening suggestions (adapted from Hammond, 1990; Hartland, 1971), and (c) forward projection (image of effective coping and gradual improvement in the future). Each patient was given a self-hypnosis tape with ego-strengthening suggestions for home practice. Outcome measures consisted of the revised Beck Depression Inventory (BDI-II) (Beck, Steer, & Brown,

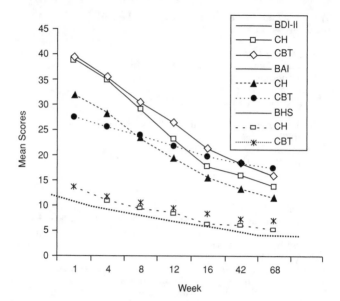

**Fig. 5.1.   Changes in BDI-II, BAI, and BHS mean scores over time for CH and CBT groups.** *Note*: Week 1, week 42, and week 68 represent baseline, 6-month, and 12-month mean scores, respectively. CH, cognitive hypnotherapy; CBT, cognitive behavior therapy; BDI-II, Beck Depression Inventory II; BAI, Beck Anxiety Index; BHS, Beck Hopelessness Scale.

1996), the Beck Anxiety Inventory (BAI) (Beck & Steer, 1993), and the Beck Hopelessness Scale (BHS) (Beck & Steer, 1993a). The inclusion criteria included *DSM-IV* (American Psychiatric Association, 1994) diagnosis of recurrent major depressive disorder and a minimum objective score of 3 on the Barber Suggestibility Scale (BSS) (Barber, 1978–1979). The measures were administered in the first, fourth, eighth, twelfth, and sixteenth sessions, and at 6-month and 12-month follow-ups.

Figure 5.1 shows the level of improvement in the two treatment groups. At the end of the 16-week treatment, the majority of the patients from both groups significantly improved compared to baseline scores. However, the CH group produced significantly larger changes in the BDI-II, $t(41) = 15.9$, $p < .001$, the BAI, $t(41) = 12.2$, $p < .001$, and the BHS, $t(41) = 12.4$, $p < .001$ scores. The improvements were maintained at 6- and 12-month follow-up. In addition, effect size calculations indicated that the CH group had a 6.03% greater reduction in depression, 5.08% greater reduction in anxiety, and 8.05% greater reduction in hopelessness above and beyond the CBT group at the termination of treatment. The effect size was maintained at 6- and 12-month follow-ups. This indicates that the depressed patients from the CH group continued to improve after the termination of treatment. We (Alladin & Alibhai, 2007) believe this is because of the utilization of the self-hypnosis tape. The patients from the CH group reported that they found it very helpful to listen to their self-hypnosis tape daily after the termination of the treatment. There was also a correlation between hypnotic suggestibility and treatment outcome. Irrespective of treatment modality, the moderate to highly susceptible subjects produced significantly more improvement than the lowly suggestible subjects. This was more apparent at the termination of treatment (week 16) and during follow-ups (weeks 42 and 68). These results clearly demonstrate that CH is equally, or even more, effective than CBT in the management of chronically depressed patients. From the results of this study, one can conclude that adding hypnosis to CBT increases the effect size of the treatment. The study met criteria for "probably efficacious" treatment and not for "well-established treatment," because the study was conducted at a single site. Arrangements are underway to have the study replicated at two independent sites.

Although the study clearly demonstrated the benefits of combining hypnotherapy with CBT in the treatment of chronic depression, it is not clear which hypnotherapeutic strategies (several hypnotherapeutic strategies were utilized) were instrumental in producing the additive change. A dismantling design is required to study the effect of each hypnotherapeutic component. However, we (Alladin & Alibhai, 2007) have discussed the possible role of the following hypnotherapeutic components: *hypnotic induction*, *ego-strengthening*, *expansion of awareness*, *positive mood induction*, *post-hypnotic suggestions*, and *self-hypnosis* in the amelioration of the depressive symptoms. In this book, CH utilizes these hypnotherapeutic components to maximize the treatment gain and reduce relapse.

## SUMMARY

This chapter discussed the clinical implications and the effectiveness of the CFMD. The order in which the techniques are presented in Part III of the book follows the sequence of intervention I have found most useful. However, the sequence of intervention described should not be regarded as invariable; the sequence must be altered to suit each individual patient. For example, if a moderately severe depressed patient is preoccupied with suicide, then the therapist should address the suicide first, then consider using First Aid for Depression (Chapter 7), rather than progressing sequentially as per the model. In the case of a depressed patient with high anxiety, hypnotherapy can be introduced prior to initiating CBT.

## REFERENCES

Alladin, A. (1994). Cognitive hypnotherapy with depression. *Journal of Cognitive Psychotherapy: An International Quarterly*, 8(4), 275–288.

Alladin, A. (2005). *Cognitive hypnotherapy for depression: An empirical investigation*. Paper presented at the American Psychological Association Annual Convention, Washington, DC.

Alladin, A. (2006). Cognitive hypnotherapy for treating depression. In R.A. Chapman (Ed.), *The clinical use of hypnosis in cognitive behavior therapy: A practitioner's casebook* (pp. 139–187). New York: Springer Publishing Company.

Alladin, A., & Alibhai, A. (2007). Cognitive hypnotherapy for depression: An empirical investigation. *International Journal of Clinical and Experimental Hypnosis*, in press.

American Psychiatric Association (1994). *Diagnostic and statistical manual of mental disorders* (4th ed.). Washington, DC: American Psychiatric Association.

Barber, T.X., & Wilson, S.C. (1978–1979). The Barber Suggestibility Scale and the Creative Imagination Scale—Experimental and clinical applications. *American Journal of Clinical Hypnosis*, 21, 85.

Beck, A.T., Rush, A.J., Shaw, B.F., & Emery, G. (1979). *Cognitive therapy of depression*. New York: Guilford.

Beck, A.T., & Steer, R.A. (1993). *Manual for the Beck Anxiety Inventory*. San Antonio TX: The Psychological Corporation, Harcourt Brace & Co.

Beck, A.T., & Steer, R.A. (1993a). *Manual for the Beck Hopelessness Scale*. San Antonio TX: The Psychological Corporation, Harcourt Brace & Co.

Beck, A.T., Steer, R.A., & Brown, K.B. (1996). *Beck Depression Inventory-II*. San Antonio TX: The Psychological Corporation, Harcourt Brace & Co.

Blackburn, I.M., Bishop, S., Glen, A.I.M., Whalley, L.G., & Christie, J.E. (1981). The efficacy of cognitive therapy in depression: A treatment trial using cognitive therapy and pharmacotherapy, each alone and in combination. *British Journal of Psychiatry*, 139, 181–189.

Chambless, D.L., & Hollon, S.D. (1998). Defining empirically supported therapies. *Journal of Consulting and Clinical Psychology*, 66, 7–18.

Gibbons, D.E. (1979). *Applied hypnosis and hyperempiria*. New York: Plenum Press.

Hammond, D.C. (Ed.) (1990). *Handbook of hypnotic suggestions and metaphors*. New York: W.W. Norton & Company.

Hartland, J. (1971). *Medical and dental hypnosis and its clinical applications* (2nd ed.). London: Bailliere Tindall.

Kovacs, M., Rush, A.J., Beck, A.T., & Hollon, S.D. (1981). Depressed out patients treated with cognitive therapy or pharmacotherapy: A one-year follow-up. *Archives of General Psychiatry*, 38, 33–39.

Simons, A.D., Garfield, S.L., & Murphy, G.E. (1984). The process of change in cognitive therapy and pharmacotherapy for depression. *Archives of General Psychiatry*, 41, 45–51.

Taylor, F.G., & Marshall, W.L. (1977). Experimental analysis of cognitive-behavioral therapy for depression. *Cognitive Therapy and Research*, 1, 59–72.

Weissman, M.M., Klerman, G.L., Prusoff, B.A., Sholomskas, D., & Padian, N. (1981). Depressed out patients: Results one year after treatment with drug and/or interpersonal psychotherapy. *Archives of General Psychiatry*, 38, 52–55.

Weissman, M.M., Prusoff, B.A., DiMascio, A., Neu, C., Goklaney, M., & Klerman, G.L. (1979). The efficacy of drugs and psychotherapy in the treatment of acute depressive episodes. *American Journal of Psychiatry*, 136, 555–558.

Williams, J.M.G. (1992). *The psychological treatment of depression*. London: Routledge.

# III

# A Comprehensive Approach to Treating Clinical Depression

# Cognitive Hypnotherapy Case Formulation

The main function of a case formulation is to devise an effective treatment plan. This chapter discusses the role of cognitive hypnotherapy case conceptualization in selecting effective and efficient treatment strategies. This approach emphasizes the role of cognitive distortions, negative self-instructions, irrational automatic thoughts and beliefs, schemas, and negative ruminations or negative self-hypnosis (NSH). Evidence suggests that matching treatment to particular patient characteristics increases outcome (Beutler, Clarkin, & Bongar, 2000). As mentioned in Chapter 4, case conceptualization is one of the most important clinical skills. By conceptualizing a case, the clinician develops a working hypothesis on how the patient's problems can be understood in terms of the circular feedback model. This understanding provides a compass or guide to understanding the treatment process. Persons (1989) posited that psychological disorders occur at two levels: *overt difficulties* and *underlying psychological mechanisms*. Overt difficulties are signs and symptoms presented by the patient that can be described in terms of beliefs, behaviors, and emotions. The manifestation and intensity of the cognitive, behavioral, or emotional symptoms are determined by the dysfunctionality of the underlying biological and psychological mechanisms. Because the focus of this book is on psychological treatment, the underlying psychological mechanisms will be examined in detail (although biological factors are also important). Negative self-schemas are considered within the cognitive hypnotherapy case formulation to represent the underlying psychological mechanisms causing the overt difficulties in depression.

How does a clinician identify the underlying mechanisms that are causing or maintaining the depressed patient's overt difficulties? And how does the clinician translate and tailor nomothetic (general) treatment protocol to the individual (idiographic) patient? To accomplish these tasks, cognitive hypnotherapy case formulation is recommended.

## RATIONALE FOR USING INDIVIDUALIZED CASE FORMULATION

Needleman (2003) views case formulation as the process of developing an explicit parsimonious understanding of patients and their problems that effectively guides treatment. Although the effectiveness of cognitive behavioral therapy (CBT) and cognitive hypnotherapy (CH) in treating depression have been empirically validated, their clinical significance levels were derived from nomothetic (general) or standardized treatment protocols studied in randomized controlled trials (RCTs). In the clinical setting, no standard treatment protocol can be applied systematically to all patients. The task of the clinician in such a setting is to translate the nomothetic findings from RCTs to idiographic or individual patient in an evidence-based way. To accomplish this task, many writers (e.g., Person, 1989; Persons & Davidson, 2001; Persons, Davidson, & Tompkins, 2001) have recommended an evidence-based case formulation approach to treatment. Persons et al. (2001) regard the evidence-based formulation-driven approach to the treatment of each individual patient as an experiment. Within this framework, treatment begins with an assessment, which generates a hypothesis about the mechanisms causing or maintaining the depression. The hypothesis is the individualized case formulation, which the therapist uses to develop an individualized treatment plan. As treatment proceeds, the therapist collects data via further assessment to evaluate the effects of the planned treatment. If it becomes evident that the treatment is not working, the therapist reformulates the case and develops a new treatment plan, which is also monitored and evaluated. Clinical work thus becomes more systematic and hypothesis-driven. Such an approach to treatment becomes principle-driven rather than delivering treatment strategies randomly or in a predetermined order.

The greatest advantage of the formulation-driven approach to clinical work is that "when the therapist encounters setbacks during the treatment process, he or she can follow a systematic strategy to make a change in treatment (consider whether a reformulation of the case might suggest some new interventions) rather than simply making hit-or-miss changes in the treatment plan" (Persons, et al., 2001, p. 14). Nevertheless, two important drawbacks to formulation-driven approach to treatment must be noted. First, individualized formulation-driven treatments have not been widely subjected to evaluation in RCTs. Second, while monitoring treatment outcome systematically, a clinician may rely on idiosyncratic or non–evidence-based formulation and treatment. To minimize clinical judgment errors and to secure solid evidence-based individualized formulation-driven treatment, Persons, et al. (2001) suggest two recommendations:

- The initial idiographic formulation should be based on strong evidence-based nomothetic formulation.
- The initial idiographic treatment plan should be based on a nomothetic protocol that has been shown to be effective in RCTs.

The CH case formulation is based on Beck's (1976) cognitive theory and therapy, Persons and colleagues' (Persons, 1989; Persons & Davidson, 2001; Persons, Davidson, & Tompkins, 2001) evidence-based formulation-driven treatment, Chapman's (Chapman, 2006) case conceptualization model of integration of CBT and hypnosis, and Alladin's (1994, 2006) cognitive-dissociative model of depression. I have adapted the CBT case formulation model utilized by Persons, et al. (2001) to develop the cognitive hypnotherapy case formulation. The cognitive hypnotherapy case formulation approach is recommended for three main reasons: (a) it provides a systematic method for individualizing treatment, (b) it allows the therapist to take an empirical approach to treatment of each case, and (c) it provides direction and evaluation during the treatment process.

## ASSUMPTIONS IN COGNITIVE HYPNOTHERAPY CASE FORMULATION

The circular feedback model of depression (CFMD) makes several assumptions about depression. For CH to be effective, the CH therapist should have a complete understanding of the depressed patient's belief systems and thought processes, and how they relate to the assumptions listed here:

1. Emotions are not produced by external events, but by the perception of the events.
2. Maladaptive emotions are produced by cognitive distortions.
3. Cognitive distortions are mediated by underlying schemas.
4. Symptoms are produced when life events activate negative schemas.
5. Negative schemas can be dormant from early life, activated by certain life events.
6. Negative rumination is considered to be a form of NSH.
7. NSH leads to dissociation of negative affect and loss of control.
8. NSH leads to the development of negative or depressive pathways.
9. Depression is caused by biopsychosocial factors.
10. Depression has many underlying risk factors, and it is usually comorbid with other disorders.

### LEVELS OF CASE FORMULATION

The individualized case formulation should include an exhaustive list of patient's problems and should describe the relationships among these problems. Exhaustive information is particularly necessary when treating depressed patients with multiple psychiatric, medical, and psychosocial problems. Patients with such profiles are usually not included in RCTs. They are, however, common in the clinical setting, so it is important to obtain an exhaustive list of problems that will help the therapist develop a working hypothesis and prioritize treatment goals. CH case formulation can occur at three different levels:

- Formulation at the case level
- Formulation at the problem or syndrome level
- Formulation at the situation level

The initial case level formulation is developed after three or four sessions of therapy. At this level, the clinician develops a conceptualization of the case as a whole. In formulation at this level, it is very important to explain the relationships among the patient's problems. Establishing the relationship among the problems helps the clinician to focus on problems that may be causing other problems. For example, depression may be caused or maintained by marital problems that merit early intervention.

Formulation at the problem or syndrome level provides a conceptualization of a particular clinical problem or syndrome, such as depressive symptoms, shoplifting, insomnia, obsessive-compulsive disorder, or bingeing and purging. The cognitive-dissociative model is used to conceptualize depression, while cognitive-behavioral theories are used to explain other associated syndromes (e.g., panic disorder). The clinician's treatment plan for the syndrome or problem depends on the formulation of the problem. For example, a patient's complaint of fatigue in response to a recent professional setback can be attributed to either abuse of hypnotics or negative thoughts ("There's no point in trying – I always fail"). Different formulations suggest different interventions.

Formulation at the situation level provides a "mini-formulation" of the patient's reactions in a particular situation in terms of cognitions, ruminations, behaviors, and affect that guides the clinician's intervention in that situation. Beck has provided the Thought Record format (see CAB Form in Chapter 8) to develop a situation-level formulation. The case-level formulation is accrued from information collected in the situation-level and problem-level formulations.

All levels of formulation provide direction for intervention. However, all formulations should be treated as hypotheses, and the clinician should constantly revise and sharpen the formulations as therapy proceeds. Moreover, a complete case formulation should also contain many other relevant components not detailed here, such as family history, medical conditions, and developmental history.

## FORMAT OF COGNITIVE HYPNOTHERAPY CASE FORMULATION

To identify the mechanisms that underlie the patient's depression, I use an eight-step case formulation, derived from the work of Persons, et al. (2001) and Ledley, Marx, and Heimberg (2005). The eight components, summarized in Table 6.1, are described in detail in the following sections. Appendix 6A supplies a template for a CH case formulation and treatment plan, and Appendix 6B provides the formulated case and treatment plan for Mary, a 29-year-old single woman with a 6-year history of recurrent major depressive disorder.

### Problem List

The problem list is an exhaustive list of the patient's main presenting problems and other relevant psychosocial issues, derived from the assessment information. Persons and Davidson (2001) recommend stating the patient's difficulties in concrete behavioral terms. The list should include any difficulties the patient

**Table 6.1.   Eight-step cognitive hypnotherapy case formulation**

1. List the major symptoms and problems in functioning.
2. Formulate a formal psychiatric diagnosis.
3. Formulate a working hypothesis.
4. Identify the precipitants and activating situations.
5. Explore the origin of negative self-schemas.
6. Summarize the working hypothesis.
7. Outline the treatment plan.
8. Identify strengths and assets and predict obstacles to treatment.

**Appendix 6A.   Cognitive hypnotherapy case formulation and treatment plan**

**Identifying information:**
Today's Date:
Name:
Age:
Gender:
Marital Status:
Ethnicity:
Occupational Status:
Living Situation:
Referred by:

**1. Problem list:**
(List all major symptoms and problems in functioning.)
Psychological/psychiatric symptoms:
Interpersonal difficulties:
Occupational problems:
Medical problems:
Financial difficulties:
Housing problems:
Legal issues:
Leisure problems:

**2. Diagnosis:**
Axis I:
Axis II:
Axis III:
Axis IV:
Axis V:

**3. Working hypothesis:**
(Hypothesize the underlying mechanism producing the listed problems.)
Assess schemas related to:
Self:
Other:
World:
Future:
Recurrent core beliefs
Rumination/NSH:
Hypnotic suggestibility:

**4. Precipitant/activating situations:**
(List triggers for current problems and establish connection between underlying mechanism and triggers of current problems.)
Triggers:
Are triggers congruent with self-schemas/rumination/self-hypnosis?

**5. Origins of core beliefs:**
(Establish origin of core beliefs from childhood's experience.)
Early adverse negative life-events:
Genetic predisposition:
History of treatment (include response):

(continued)

**Appendix 6A.    (Continued)**

**6. Summary of working hypothesis**
1.
2.
3.

**7. Treatment plan:**
1.
2.
3.
4.
Modality:
Frequency:
Interventions:
Adjunct Therapies:
Obstacles:

**8. Strengths and Assets:**
(Based on the formulation, predict obstacles to treatment that
    may arise.)
1.
2.
3.

**Appendix 6B.    Cognitive hypnotherapy case formulation
and treatment plan: A completed example**

**Identifying information:**
Today's Date: *June 15, 2005* Name: *Mary*
Age: *29 years old*
Gender: *Female*
Marital Status: *Single*
Ethnicity: *White Caucasian*
Occupational Status: *Administrative Assistant*
Living Situation: *Lives on her own in a rented apartment*
Referred by: *Dr. Spock, Psychiatrist*

**Problem list:**
(List all major symptoms and problems in functioning.)
Psychological/psychiatric symptoms:
*Depressed, lacking motivation, unfocused, disturbed sleep, tired,
lacking energy, and difficult concentrating. At times she feels
suicidal, but has no intent or plan. She feels angry and fearful about
the world. She always feels a sense of inner tension and can't
unwind or relax.*

Interpersonal difficulties:
*She is socially isolated, avoids friends and social events. She has
good social skills and several close women friends. She has never
dated seriously, but she wants to marry and have children. Her
friends from her office have, on several occasions, arranged for her to
meet men, but she always declined their offers at the last minute.
She believes she will never marry because she feels uncomfortable
meeting men.*

(continued)

**Appendix 6B.   (Continued)**

Occupational problems:
*She works as an administrative assistant in a small office consisting of six other women. She does not dislike her job, but she would like to hold a more responsible job in the future. However, she believes she is not bright enough to go to college for further training.*

Medical problems:
*None*
Financial difficulties:
*None*
Housing problems:
*None*
Legal issues:
*None*
Leisure problems:
*She avoids going out because she feels unsafe. She spends her leisure time in her apartment reading romantic novels or watching television.*

**2. Diagnosis:**
Axis I: *Major Depressive Disorder, Recurrent, Moderate*
Axis II: *Avoidant personality traits*
Axis III: *None*
Axis IV: *Socially isolated, lonely.*
Axis V: *GAF score = 50*

**3. Working hypothesis:**
(Hypothesize the underlying mechanism producing the listed problems.)
Assess schemas related to:
Self:
*"I am abnormal and weird because I can't go out and meet people."*
*"I am a coward and a loser."*
*"I am ugly and unattractive, no one will like me."*
*"I am a freak, I can't even date."*
Other:
*"You can't depend on others, people are bad and selfish, they always want to hurt you."*
World:
*"The world is scary and no one is there to protect you."*
*"I hate the world."*
Future:
*"My future is uncertain and bleak."*
*"I see myself being lonely and isolated for the rest of my life."*
*"At times, I feel life is not worth living."*
Recurrent core beliefs:
*"I am abnormal, there's something wrong with me and I will never be normal."*
Rumination/NSH:
*She ruminates with the belief that she is not normal and often has the image of being isolated and lonely for the rest of her life, and there is no one to care for her. She reports having a good imagination, but she tends to focus more on negative thoughts.*
Hypnotic suggestibility:
*She scored maximum on the Barer Suggestibility Scale.*

(continued)

## Appendix 6B. (Continued)

### 4. Precipitant/activating situations
(List triggers for current problems and establish connection between underlying mechanism and triggers of current problems.)

Triggers:
*Watching other women dating or getting married. One of the women from her office got engaged, and this triggered her depressive episode. Other activating events include attending special social functions such as wedding, Christmas party, or not able to go on a date.*

Are triggers congruent with self-schemas/rumination/self-hypnosis?
*The triggers activate her self-schema of being abnormal or defective.*

### 5. Origins of core beliefs
(Establish origin of core beliefs from childhood's experience.)
Early adverse negative life-events:
*She was brought up in a very hostile and stressful environment. Her father was a gambler and an alcoholic. On many occasions, she witnessed her father being physically aggressive toward her mother, who never confronted her husband or tried to get out of the relationship, or sought help to sort out her domestic problems. He constantly undermined Mary and called her "stupid" and "a whore." Mary was scared and frightened of her father, and often used to have nightmares about her father killing her and her mother. The most traumatic experience for Mary was when her father got her out of the shower naked to switch the TV off. Mary left the TV on while she was having a shower. She was 11 years old. Mary learned to be scared of men, and she became passive, fragile, and unassertive like her mother.*

Genetic predisposition:
*Mary's mother and grandmother have a history of major depressive disorder. Mary reported that, like her, her mother too has a tendency to think very negatively about everything.*

History of treatment (include response):
*Followed up by a psychiatrist for 3 years. Tried several antidepressant medications, but none has worked for her. Also seen a mental health therapist in the community for counseling. She derived support from the counseling but did not improve her symptoms significantly.*

### 6. Summary of working hypothesis:
*Whenever Mary faced a special social event such as an engagement or a wedding, she felt uncomfortable and, at times, she had to leave the function. Such events revived her schema that she is weird, abnormal, defective, and a failure. From her abusive father she learned that she is defective and a failure, and from her mother's passivity she learned that she is incapable of taking actions. Hence she avoided anxious situations and never learned to cope with her anxiety and discomfort, thus maintained her negative schema and associated depressive affect.*

### 7. Strengths and assets:
*Stable lifestyle; bright; excellent social skills; has friends.*

(continued)

**Appendix 6B.   (Continued)**

**8. Treatment plan**

Goals (Measures):

1. *Reduce depressive symptoms via BDI-II, procrastination via log of activities.*
2. *Increase ability to prioritize and organize work and at home.*
3. *Find a more satisfying job (measured directly).*
4. *Increase time spent with friends (measured via number of contacts).*
5. *Begin dating in an effort to meet husband (measured via number of dates).*
6. *Increase assertiveness (measured via log of assertive behaviors).*

Modality:
*Individual cognitive hypnotherapy.*

Frequency:
*Weekly for 10 weeks.*

Interventions:
*Teach the formulation (to provide rationale for interventions).*
*Activity scheduling (work tasks, socializing, dating, job search).*
*Cognitive restructuring (RET-Worksheet, behavioral experiments).*
*Assertive training.*
*Schema change interventions.*

Adjunct Therapies:
*Medication will be considered an option if she does not respond to cognitive-hypnotherapy.*

Obstacles:
*Procrastination, unassertiveness, "I'm incapable of succeeding."*

---

is having in any of the following domains:

- Psychological/psychiatric symptoms
- Interpersonal difficulties
- Occupational problems
- Medical symptoms
- Financial difficulties
- Housing problems
- Legal problems
- Leisure activities

Compiling a comprehensive list of problems ensures that important problems are not overlooked, while simultaneously ensuring that the therapist does not become overwhelmed with a patient's multitudinous problems. Moreover, the list may show "themes" in the causal relationships among problems and help to develop working hypotheses.

### Diagnosis

An accurate diagnosis of depression provides information for the initial formulation of hypotheses and for formulating a treatment plan. It is recommended that a formal diagnostic nomenclature such as the *DSM-IV-TR* (American Psychiatric Association, 2000) is used to make a diagnosis. An accurate diagnosis also facilitates differentiating the subtype of depression and co-morbid disorders. As discussed in Chapter 2, Beck (Beck, et al., 1987) has provided empirical evidence to his *content-specificity* hypothesis, which maintains that although negativity is common to all emotional disorders, each disorder has its own specific set of cognitive distortions. Therefore an accurate diagnosis provides schema hypotheses. For example, it is known that depressed patients hold typical negative schemas about themselves, others, the world, and the future, and therefore a diagnosis of depression will guide the therapist to look for depressive schemas hypotheses. A psychiatric diagnosis also serves as a link to RCTs and empirically supported nomothetic treatment interventions (Persons, et al., 2001).

## Working Hypotheses

The working hypothesis is central to case formulation, and it can be subdivided into four headings: schema, activating events, origins, and summary.

### Schemas

Schemas or core beliefs are deep cognitive structures that people have held for much of their lives, and which are activated across a wide range of situations. These schemas have a profound influence on how people feel, appraise situations, and see themselves and the world (Needleman, 2003). The therapist attempts to offer hypotheses about the core beliefs that may be causing or maintaining the difficulties identified in the problem list. The CFMD depression emphasizes the importance of (a) understanding the patient's beliefs about self, others, world, and future (cognitive triad), (b) the extent to which a patient ruminates and indulges in NSH, and (c) the capacity of a depressed patient to experience hypnotic trance. Therefore, within the CH case formulation, maladaptive cognitions, negative ruminations, negative self-hypnosis, and hypnotic suggestibility are routinely assessed. Appendix 6B provides Mary's negative views on several cognitive domains. Although depressed patients may have multiple negative beliefs, they tend to ruminate with one or two core beliefs. According to Nolen-Hoeksema (1991), rumination represents a process of perseverative attention that is directed to specific, mainly internal, content (see Chapter 4). For example, a depressed person may become focused on her negative affect, the causes of the negative feeling, and the consequences of the depressed mood. In the case of Mary, her core beliefs centered around, *"I am abnormal, there's something wrong with me and I will never be normal."* She ruminated on the negative self-suggestions that she is not normal and that she will be isolated and lonely for the rest of her life, with no one to care for her (see Appendix 6B). Such perseverative attention can be regarded as a form of NSH. Moreover, negative schemas and negative beliefs add more vitality to NSH, which serves to counter positive suggestions from self or others. The cognitive-dissociative model conceptualizes that patients who are highly susceptible to hypnosis are more likely to be syncretically involved in their ruminations. This is the reason for assessing NSH and hypnotic suggestibility within the CH case formulation. Although the concept of hypnotic suggestibility is controversial, it is my belief that patients who score low on standard hypnotic suggestibility scales may not derive maximum benefit from hypnotherapy. For such patients, relaxation or imagery training can be substituted for hypnosis. The standard tests not only indicate which patient is highly suggestible, but the assessment also serves as an experiment to discover what kinds of suggestions the depressed patient responds to. Such information guides the therapist in crafting and delivering congruent induction, and hypnotic and posthypnotic suggestions. For example, if a depressed patient obtained his highest score on "arm heaviness" and low score on "arm levitation" on the Barber Suggestibility Scale, then it would be more appropriate to use suggestions of heaviness for hypnotic induction, deepening, and posthypnotic suggestions regarding self-hypnosis.

## Precipitants and Activating Situations

In this stage of case conceptualization, the therapist specifies external events that activate schemas to produce symptoms and problems. External events can be categorized into two classes: *precipitating events* and *activating situations*. Precipitating events are large-scale, molar events that trigger a depressive episode. For example, a depressive episode can be precipitated in a young adult who leaves home to go to the university. Activating situations refer to smaller-scale events that precipitate negative affect or maladaptive behaviors. Often these smaller-scale activating situations can trigger the same schema activated by precipitating events. For example, the student who left home felt lonely while studying in his room at the university residence. In this example, both the precipitating event (leaving home) and the activating situation (alone in his room) triggered the same schema ("I'm weak, I can't cope").

There are several important reasons for assessing external events and situations. First, since the cognitive theory of depression attributes symptoms to the activation of underlying schema, and not to external events or intrapsychic events, there ought to be a match between the patient's schema and the external events that activated the schema. It is important for the therapist to have a good understanding of the relationship between external events and core beliefs, because the focus of CBT is to change the schema. Second, there are times when a connection cannot be made between external events and core beliefs because the schema remains unconscious. CBT is not designed to explore deep unconscious cognitions. This limitation of CBT is compensated by the inclusion of hypnotherapy in CH. Hypnotherapy provides several effective techniques for eliciting and changing unconscious schemas. Third, although the focus of CBT is on core beliefs and not on external events, external events can be problematic to some patients. For example, an abusive relationship may create situations in which safety for a partner may be compromised. Identification of such problematic events can provide important information while formulating intervention strategies. Four, at times it is beneficial for patients to change their situations rather than simply changing their reactions to the situations. For example, the young man who went to university can share his room with another student to avoid loneliness. The foregoing clearly illustrates that depression is a complex disorder, involving multiple factors; hence, treatment should be broadened to deal with all the triggering, maintaining, and risk factors. Mary's main triggering factors seem to be special occasions such as dating, engagement, and weddings (see Appendix 6B).

## Origins

In this section of the case formulation, the therapist draws information from the patient's early history to understand how the patient might have learned her problematic schema. It is recommended that the therapist summarizes this understanding with a simple statement or by providing a brief description of one or two poignant incidents that capture the patient's early experience. For example, as a child, Mary was continually punished by her parents for playing outside her house, while her brother got away with it. The parents pointed out to her that girls are not allowed to play outside the house, because the girl's place is in the home. Consequently, Mary learned that "I am not important, I am inferior." Information about modeling experiences (e.g., Mary learned from her parents to treat boys and girls differently) and failure to learn certain important skills or behaviors (e.g., Mary was afraid to question her parents and did not learn to be assertive) can also be included in this section. It is also important to obtain a history of mental illness in the family. Although depression is not a hereditary illness, within the biopsychosicial (diathesis-stress) model, biological factors serve as diathesis to depression. Because of the biological diathesis, a person may be predisposed to develop problematic schemas. Mary's mother had a long history of major depressive disorder, and Mary had a pessimistic view of life since childhood. Her negative self-schemas were molded (a) by the way she was treated by her father and (b) by a negative experience (an incident in which her father forced her out of the shower naked to switch off the TV, which she left on) that she cannot get out of her mind (see under Origins of Core Beliefs in Appendix 6B).

## Summary of Working Hypothesis

This section forms the heart of the case formulation. Here the therapist describes how the components of the working hypothesis (schema, precipitants and activating situations, and origins) interact with each other to produce the depressive symptoms and the problems listed on the patient's problem list. The summary of the working hypothesis can be described either verbally or using a diagram with arrows linking the components on the formulation (see Persons & Davidson, 2001). Mary's negative schema, originating from her abusive father, is triggered by special social events such as engagement parties and weddings, leading to the triggering and maintenance of anxiety and depression (see Appendix 6B).

## Strengths and Assets

Gathering information about the patient's strengths and assets (e.g., social support, good social skills, financial resources, stable lifestyle, good physical health, etc.) serves several purposes. It helps the therapist develop a working hypothesis, it enhances the treatment plan by integrating the patient's strengths and assets, and it can assist in the determination of realistic treatment goals. Mary's strengths and assets include above-average intelligence, stable lifestyle, excellent social life, and having several close friends.

**Treatment Plan**

Although the treatment plan is not part of the case formulation, it is included here to stress the point that the treatment plan is based directly on the case formulation. One of the main reasons for CH case formulation is to guide the therapist in selecting effective and efficient interventions. Evidence suggests that therapeutic success is increased when interventions are matched to particular patient characteristics (Beutler, Clarkin, & Bongar, 2000). The treatment plan of the formulation has six components including goals, modality, frequency, interventions, adjunct therapies, and obstacles. Each of these components is described in detail.

*Goals*

The therapist and the patient collaborate to develop treatment goals to deal with the symptoms and problems listed on the problem list. Most patients seek treatment to address one or two important or distressing problems, rather than trying to solve all their problems. It is therefore important for the therapist and the patient to be in complete agreement about the treatment goals. It is unlikely that treatment will be successful if there is disagreement between the therapist and the patient regarding the treatment goals or problem list.

Treatment goals must be stated concretely, and progress toward the goals must be measured. Specifying treatment goals in clear, concrete statements facilitates therapeutic work. For example, a vague goal statement such as "Jane will get better" is not concrete enough to provide guidance for setting specific goals for the treatment sessions. But a concrete statement such as "Jane will reduce her depressive symptoms," provides clear guidance to setting agendas for the treatment sessions. Moreover, setting concrete goals facilitates outcome measurement. Measurement of progress toward the treatment goal provides a tool for the therapist to track down progress. If the initial treatment plan does not work, it will be necessary to revise the case formulation and the treatment plan. For each formulated goal, it is advisable to use at least one measure to monitor treatment progress. Measures can range from simple counts (e.g., keeping a count of daily activities, number of panic attacks) to self-rating measures (e.g., Beck Depression Inventory). As recommended by Persons, et al. (2001), I routinely ask my depressed patients to complete the revised Beck Depression Inventory (BDI-II) (Beck, Steer, & Brown, 1996), the Beck Anxiety Inventory (BAI) (Beck & Steer, 1993), and the Beck Hopelessness Scale (BHS) (Beck & Steer, 1993a) prior to each therapy session to monitor their weekly progress. The scores from these three self-rating measures can be plotted on a graph to track the patient's progress with depressive and anxiety symptoms. The graph provides a visual representation of the patient's progress. Idiographic measures such as self-monitoring can also be tailored to assess the patient's problems.

Changes in dysfunctional thinking can also be monitored by utilizing any of these three self-rating assessment tools suggested by Nezu, Nezu, and Lombardo (2004):

- *Automatic Thought Questionnaire-Revised* (Kendall, Howard, & Hays, 1989): This self-rating questionnaire measures both negative and positive self-statements related to depression (e.g., "I'm worthless").
- *Cognitive Triad Inventory* (Beckham, Leber, Watkins, Boyer, & Cook, 1986): This self-rating measure is designed to assess aspects of Beck's (Beck, et al., 1979) cognitive triad (see Chapter 2).
- *Dysfunctional Attitude Scale* (Weissman & Beck, 1978): This self-report inventory measures depression-related dysfunctional cognitions.

### Modality

Specify the treatment approach utilized (e.g., individual CH).

### Frequency

State the frequency of treatment sessions required (e.g., once a week).

### Interventions

The interventions proposed in the treatment plan are based directly on the CH case formulation. Most importantly, they are related to the deficits described in the working hypothesis, they address some of the problems identified on the problem list, and they facilitate the accomplishment of the goals (Persons, Davidson, & Tompkins, 2001). For example, activity scheduling will be a logical intervention for a depressed man who is passive and inactive and spends most of his time staying in bed in his apartment. A depressed person who is lacking social skills because of social inhibition, based on the belief that he is not liked by anyone, will benefit from social skills training. McKnight, Nelson, Hayes, and Jarrett (1984), from a series of single-case studies, have provided evidence that interventions tailored to depressed patient's deficits are most beneficial. They found depressed patients with social skills deficits to benefit most from social skills training, while those with cognitive distortions benefited most from cognitive restructuring. It is therefore recommended that therapists use evidence-based interventions to strengthen the empirical foundation of CH for depression.

### Adjunct Therapies

Most depressed patients seen in clinical practice have multitudinous problems and comorbid conditions. Very often adjunctive interventions such as pharmacotherapy, family therapy, and substance abuse counseling may be required. It is recommended that the therapist be alert to the depressed patient's complex needs and facilitate adjunctive interventions as necessary. If Mary's depressive symptoms are not reduced via CH, antidepressant medication can be considered as an adjunct treatment.

### Obstacles

The final component of the treatment plan uses the information from the case formulation to predict difficulties that might arise in the therapeutic relationship or in the course of the therapy. Certain items from problem list, such as interpersonal difficulties, financial problems, medical problems, or occupational difficulties, can alert the therapist to those factors that may interfere with therapeutic progress. Early awareness of potential obstacles helps the patient and therapist cope more effectively with the problems when they arise.

### SUMMARY

The CH case formulation provides a model for selecting effective treatment strategies for individual (idiographic) depressed patients from the available nomothetic research literature. This model stresses the role of multiple risk factors in the onset, exacerbation, and maintenance of depression. By conceptualizing a case, the therapist develops a working hypothesis on how the patient's problems can be understood in terms of the circular feedback model. This understanding provides a framework for understanding the treatment process. Within this model, treatment begins with an assessment, which generates a hypothesis about the mechanisms causing or maintaining the depression. The hypothesis is the individualized case formulation, which the therapist uses to develop the individualized treatment plan. As treatment proceeds, the therapist collects data via further assessment to evaluate the effects of the planned treatment. Chapters 7 to 15 describe various treatment strategies within the CH framework. If it becomes evident that the treatment is not working, the therapist reformulates the case and develops a new treatment plan, which is also monitored and evaluated. Within this framework, clinical work becomes systematic and hypothesis-driven, rather than delivering treatment strategies randomly or in a predetermined order. Appendix 6A provides a template for CH case formulation, and Appendix 6B offers a completed example of a formulated case.

### REFERENCES

Alladin, A. (1994). Cognitive hypnotherapy with depression. *Journal of Cognitive Psychotherapy: An International Quarterly*, 8(4), 275–288.

Alladin, A. (2006). Cognitive hypnotherapy for treating depression. In R.A. Chapman (Ed.), *The clinical use of hypnosis in cognitive behavior therapy: A practitioner's casebook* (pp. 139–187). New York: Springer Publishing Company.

American Psychiatric Association (2000). *Diagnostic and statistical manual of mental disorders* (4th ed., revised). Washington, DC: American Psychiatric Association.

Beck, A. (1976). *Cognitive therapy and emotional disorders*. New York: International University Press.

Beck, A.T., Brown, G., Steer, R.A., Eidelson, J.I., & Riskind, J.H. (1987). Differentiating anxiety and depression: A test of the cognitive-content-specificity hypothesis. *Journal of Abnormal Psychology*, 96, 179–183.

Beck, A.T., Rush, A.J., Shaw, B.F., & Emery, G. (1979). *Cognitive therapy of depression*. New York: Guilford Press.

Beck, A.T., & Steer, R.A. (1993). *Beck Anxiety Inventory*. San Antonio, TX: Harcourt Brace.

Beck, A.T., & Steer, R.A. (1993a). *Beck Hopelessness Scale*. San Antonio, TX: Harcourt Brace.

Beck, A.T., Steer, R.A., & Brown, K.B. (1996). *The Beck Depression Inventory–Revised*. San Antonio, TX: Harcourt Brace.

Beckham, E.E., Leber, W.R., Watkins, J.T., Boyer, J.L., & Cook, J.B. (1986). Development of an instrument to measure Beck's cognitive triad: The Cognitive Triad Inventory. *Journal of Consulting and Clinical Psychology*, 54, 566–567.

Beutler, L.E., Clarkin, J.E., & Bongar, B. (2000). *Guidelines for the systematic treatment of the depressed patient*. New York: Oxford University Press.

Chapman, R.A. (2006). Case conceptualization model for integration of cognitive behavior therapy and hypnosis. In R.A. Chapman (Ed.), *The clinical use of hypnosis in cognitive behavior therapy: A practitioner's casebook* (pp. 71–98). New York: Springer Publishing Company.

Kendall, P.C., Howard, B.L., & Hays, R.C. (1989). Self-referent speech and psychopathology: The balance of positive and negative thinking. *Cognitive Therapy and Research*, 13, 583–598.

Ledley, D.R., Marx, B.P., & Heimberg, R.G. (2005). *Making cognitive-behavioral therapy work: Clinical process for new practitioners*. The Guilford Press: New York.

McKnight, D.L., Nelson, R.O., Hayes, S.C., & Jarrett, R.B. (1984). Importance of treating individually assessed response classes in the amelioration of depression. *Behavior Therapy*, 15, 315–335.

Needleman, L.D. (2003). Case conceptualization in preventing and responding to therapeutic difficulties. In R.L. Leahy (Ed.), *Roadblocks in cognitive-behavioral therapy: Transforming challenges into opportunities for change* (pp. 3–23). New York: The Guilford Press.

Nezu, A.M., Nezu, C.M., & Lombardo, E. (2004). *Cognitive-behavioral case formulation and treatment design: A problem-solving approach*. New York: Springer Publishing Company.

Nolen-Hoeksema, S. (1991). Responses to depression and their effects on the duration of depressive episodes. *Journal of Abnormal Psychology*, 100, 569–582.

Persons, J.B. (1989). *Cognitive therapy in practice: A case formulation approach*. New York: Norton.

Persons, J.B., & Davidson, J. (2001). Cognitive-behavioral case formulation. In K. Dobson (Ed.), *Handbook of cognitive-behavioral therapies* (pp. 86–110). New York: Guilford Press.

Persons, J.B., Davidson, J., & Tompkins, M.A. (2001). *Essential components of cognitive-behavior therapy for depression*. Washington, DC: American Psychological Association.

Weissman, A.N., & Beck, A.T. (1978). *Development and validation of the Dysfunctional Attitude Scale: A preliminary investigation*. Paper presented at the meeting of the Association for the Advancement of Behavior Therapy, Chicago.

# First Aid For Depression

First Aid for Depression is an innovative brief clinical intervention for dealing with acute symptoms of depression. When faced
with a stressor, depressed patients tend to become overwhelmed
with feelings of low mood, hopelessness, and a sense of pessimism.
Any immediate relief from these feelings provides a sense of hope,
promotes positive expectancy of treatment, and strengthens the
therapeutic alliance. Overlade (1986) described a First Aid technique for producing immediate relief from the depressive mood.
The technique utilizes ventilation, education, alteration in posture, and active imagery to reduce the depressive affect. The
importance of the imaginal processes has been increasingly recognized in the clinical field, and numerous imagery techniques are
utilized in the treatment of various medical and psychiatric disorders (Sheikh, 2003). Velton (1968) and Sirota and Schwartz (1982)
demonstrated that different affective states can be induced and
altered by various imagery procedures. Schultz (1978, 1984, 2003)
provided empirical evidence that directed (aggressive, socially
gratifying, and positive) imagery can break the "depressive loop"
and produce temporary relief in depressed psychiatric patients.
Similarly, Burtle (1975) produced immediate changes in the level
of depression in eight depressed patients with psychomotor retardation by providing positive imagery training. These findings
clearly demonstrate that directed imagery can help severely depressed patients reduce their level of depression for brief periods
of time.

The First Aid technique is particularly indicated when the depression is of recent onset and the precipitant is clearly identified
as accounting for the escalation of the depressed mood. This technique will not be appropriate for chronic depression and where
depression is considered to be secondary to substance abuse or
pathological conditions. I (Alladin, 1989, 1992, 1992a, 1994, 2006;
Alladin & Heap, 1991) have expanded this technique into seven
phases:

- Ventilation
- Education
- Adopting antidepressive posture
- Forcing a smile
- Imagining a "funny face"
- Playing a "happy mental tape"
- Conditioning to a cue

The First Aid Technique for depression is described and illustrated by a Case Example: Patty, a 37-year-old housewife, was
in therapy with me for about 6 months for dysthymic disorder.
She did very well with cognitive hypnotherapy (CH), so she was

discharged after twelve sessions. Eight months after discharge, Patty arranged for an urgent appointment to see me. She had an acute situational depression precipitated by her husband's unjustified anger and very cutting remarks. Patty is married to Brent, a very ambitious and workaholic business man. Brent has a tendency to undermine psychological difficulties; his philosophy is that one should be able to lead a productive and successful life in this world if one chooses to and works hard to get it. He finds it hard to tolerate people who feels depressed and "mope about." Patty, on the other hand, is very sensitive to people with emotional problems, and she strongly believes that in a marital relationship one should be able to communicate freely and be able to express one's feelings easily. Although Brent was supportive of Patty while she was depressed and undergoing psychotherapy, he sincerely believes that Patty can make a greater difference to her life "if she gives up her pessimistic and gloomy views of life."

Patty became very depressed because Brent accused her of "always moping" and being "stupid" and "useless." Patty and Brent have two children (Becky, 6 and Adam, 10) from their 12-year marriage. Recently Adam was having some difficulties at school; he was not attentive in class and was oppositional to his teacher. Matters came to a head when Mr. Smith, the principal of the school, telephoned Patty to report that Adam had been swearing at his teacher. He is thinking of suspending Adam from school and wanted to meet with the parents urgently before making the final decision. Because Brent was out of town on business, Patty went to meet with the principal. Patty convinced Mr. Smith to give Adam a chance since it was his first offense, and Patty promised that she and her husband would keep a close eye on Adam. Although the situation was satisfactorily resolved, Patty started to feel guilty that it might be her fault that Adam has been presenting behavioral problems at school. Patty became so upset that she called her husband out of town to communicate her distress. Brent was in the middle of a tough business negotiation when Patty called, so he reassured her that he would call back as soon as the meeting was over. Patty expressed anger that she could not talk to her husband whenever she wishes and stated that he does not care for the family and is more interested in his business. An hour later, Brent called and expressed his anger and frustration at Patty. Brent indicated that she is selfish, useless, and unable to resolve the slightest difficulty in his absence, and he could not understand why she was making such a big deal about Adam when the matter was resolved. Following the telephone conversation, Patty became very upset and started to ruminate on the belief that she is useless and incompetent. She was not able to sleep that night, so the next day she arranged for her appointment with me.

## VENTILATION PHASE

At this stage, the patient is encouraged to ventilate the distressing feelings precipitated by a crisis. Patty was encouraged to talk about the events that led to her despair, particularly about the "unfair" accusations and "hurtful things" Brent said to her. The ventilation of her anger, frustration, resentment, and hurt was uncritically accepted, although occasionally questions were interjected to separate facts from conjectures and suspicions.

## EDUCATION PHASE

At this stage, the patient is provided a scientific explanation of why some people get acutely depressed due to social factors. The educational focus is not so much based on scientific information, but to provide an explanation that makes sense to the patient. Providing a plausible explanation for the amplification of the depressive affect (a) validates the patient's emotional reaction, (b) reduces guilt for feeling depressed, and (c) provides a conceptual framework for instituting practical strategies for reducing the depressive affect.

Patty was provided with the explanation that emotions represent primitive mammalian responses that can be substantiated and perpetuated by intellectual reasoning. When deeply depressed, humans and primates have the tendency to adopt the same "tucking reflex," that is, the shoulders roll forward, the chin and the gaze incline downward, and the arms droop limply. At this point, especially when emotionally hurt, one cannot relinquish the depressive feeling because the human intellect validates the hurt and substantiates the right to feel depressed. Moreover, the tucking reflex produces biological negative affect, thus rendering it more difficult to alter the depressive affect simply through intellectual reasoning. However, a conscious decision to alter the tucking reflex by adopting an antidepressive posture can encourage the intellect to search for reasons to feel better.

Patient education also involves forging a link between emotion and depression. It was pointed out to Patty that the tucking reflex serves a protective function in both humans and animals. In animals, the tucking reflex provides a closing posture that serves to protect the vital organs, and it communicates a posture of capitulation to prevent further attack from a dominant animal. For example, if two monkeys are fighting for territory, the losing monkey adopts a tucking reflex to protect himself from further injury. The posture communicates to the dominant monkey that his opponent has been subdued and there is no need for further fighting. This is true of humans as well. When an infant is chided by an adult, he instinctively drops his chin and extends his lower lip in a pout, and the adult responds by easing the intensity of criticism. This experience is reinforced and, gradually, the child learns that by adopting the tucking reflex and looking penitent he can ward off criticism from dominant adults. However, it not very helpful to maintain the depressive posture for too long because this prolongs the feeling of despair and may not continue to serve as a defense. Patty listened intently. She now understands why it is sometimes useful to be depressed, but she also realizes that at a certain point it is important to break away from the depressive posture.

## ADOPTING ANTIDEPRESSIVE POSTURE PHASE

Stages three to seven can be carried out under hypnosis if the person is susceptible to hypnosis. Following the ventilation and education phases, patients are usually in a hypnoidal state. (When seeing a patient for the first time, if I am not aware of the patient's hypnotic capacity, I will not induce hypnosis or even suggest its use. I have found this procedure to work equally well without hypnosis.) Patty is very susceptible to hypnosis, and she enjoys the hypnotic modality, so I chose to use it.

Now that Patty has some insight into her depression, she was ready to adopt the antidepressive posture:

*Therapist:* Now that you know that depression is a body response, you can let it go. It is easy to let go of your depression. The most difficult part is deciding to let it go. If you are really feeling down, and a friend tries to cheer up, you will get really mad because you would think they don't understand your depression. But now that you know that depression is a body response, and your intellect tells you to feel depressed, perhaps you will able to do something to ease your depression. Would you like to do this?

*Patty:* Yes.

*Therapist:* I am going to show you how to adopt an antidepressive posture, and I will help you to get the heavy weight off your head. But first, just make yourself comfortable in the chair and close your eyes. Take a deep breath. Hold it. Now, let go .... Now I am going to count one to ten, when I reach the count of ten you will drift into a deep, deep hypnotic sleep.

At the count of ten Patty, went into a deep trance.

*Therapist:* While you are relaxing, I am going to stand behind your chair and hold your head in my hand. Is this OK?

Patty agreed. (In the case of a patient who does not agree, the therapist can use imagery instead: imagining the head is like a heavy bag full of sand with a hole punctured in it to allow the sand to trickle out. As the sands trickle out, the head gets lighter.)

*Therapist:* Now allow the weight of your head to go into my hands. Imagine you head getting lighter as all the weight of your head goes into my hands. You feel your head is becoming light...lighter...and lighter...you feel your head is becoming detached...light and detached...soon you will feel your head is completely detached. Let me know when your head feels detached by raising your 'Yes finger.'

Patty was primed to give ideomotor signals by raising her fingers. The "Yes" finger went up.

*Therapist:* Now I am going to give you back your head, leaving all the weight behind...Does your head feel light?

*Patty:* (The "Yes" finger went up.)

*Therapist:* Now I am going to show you how to adopt an antidepressive posture. I want you to imagine you are standing in front of Buckingham Palace, watching the guard on duty in front of the gate. Can you imagine it?

*Patty:* (Patty signaled "Yes.")

*Therapist:* Imagine you are pretending to be the guard on duty. Just pretend...raise your head high up...your shoulders broad and square...yours arms strong and straight by your side, with the gun in one of your hands...Can you imagine this?

Patty signaled "Yes" again.

*Therapist:* As you pretend to be the guard on duty, notice that you feel strong and straight... strong and straight.

Although still sitting in the chair, Patty's posture changed: her head went up, her shoulders broadened and squared, and her arms were held straight by her sides.

*Therapist:* Do you feel strong and straight?
The "Yes" finger went up; Patty was no longer "tucked in." She was holding her head up, adopting an antidepressive posture.

## FORCING A SMILE PHASE

Once the patient has adopted an antidepressive posture, the patient is encouraged to smile. Smiling is paradoxical to depression.

*Therapist:* Now imagine looking in a mirror and forcing yourself to smile. It is not natural to smile when you are distressed, so you have to force yourself to smile.

Patty started to smile after a short while. As she started to smile, her facial muscles relaxed and she appeared less depressed.

## IMAGINING A "FUNNY FACE" PHASE

In this phase, the therapist attempts to create a social image.

*Therapist:* Now I want you to remember a funny face. This can be a person you remember from long ago who made you laugh. When you imagine this person, there is something about this person's face or the way the person talks that makes you laugh. Just remember this person and the way the person made you laugh.

After a while Patty started to smile more naturally, then she started to laugh.

## PLAYING A "HAPPY MENTAL TAPE" PHASE

During this phase, the patient is regressed to a happy time.

*Therapist:* Now I would like you to imagine a happy time in your life, a happy memory or a happy place? Go back in time and place to a happy time in your life.

Pause. Patty nods.

*Therapist:* Now play this happy tape in your mind.
Patty progressively became more relaxed and appeared happy.

## CUE CONDITIONING PHASE

At this stage, the patient is given posthypnotic suggestions for producing relief from depression. To facilitate this, the patient is conditioned to a cue word.

*Therapist:* From now on, whenever you feel upset or depressed and do not want to feel that feeling, you can get rid of it by thinking of the word BUBBLE. When you think of BUBBLE, you will be able to remember all the details of this exercise, and you will feel much better, more optimistic.

Patty felt much better at the end of the session. She was no longer upset or distressed, and she was energized.

I have been using the First Aid for Depression with my depressed patients for over 15 years. I have noticed a dramatic alteration of the depressive affect in most of my patients who undergo the procedure, although the positive effect was reported to last for about 1 to 4 hours only. This alteration of the depressive affect, although transitory, instills hope and positive expectancy, and prepares the depressive patient for the next stage of CH. Gold and his colleagues (Jarvinen & Gold, 1981; Gold, Jarvinen, & Teague, 1982; also see review by Schultz, 2003) have extended the work of Schultz (1978) and studied the intermediate and long-term effects of directed imagery on symptoms amelioration in depressed patients. They monitored the immediate and long-term changes in level of depression of 53 mildly to moderately depressed female undergraduate students who practiced either neutral, positive, or self-generated positive imagery at least twice daily for 2 weeks, or who were assigned to a no-treatment control group. After 2 weeks, the students using the three imagery conditions reported lower scores on the Beck Depression Inventory (BDI) scale than did the no-treatment group. Students who produced more vivid imagery enjoyed greater therapeutic benefit. At 6-month follow-up, the students from both the treatment and no-treatment groups reported no significant differences in their level of depression. Nevertheless, 57% of the students from the three imagery groups, compared with 13% from the no-treatment group, reported a change in mood as result of the study. Further evidence that directed imagery procedures can reduce both self-reported and behavioral indices of depression comes from studies of mental health center patients (Lipsky, Kassinove, & Miller, 1980), adolescent delinquent girls (Reardon & Tossi, 1977), and psychiatric depressed patients (Burtle, 1976; Schultz, 1978). These studies clearly indicate the beneficial effects of directed imagery on mood, although the benefits appeared to diminish gradually over time. These findings are not surprising, because depression is a complex disorder, and it is unlikely that a single modality such as directed imagery is likely to produce lasting improvement. However, it is noteworthy that directed positive imagery does produce a significant reduction in negative mood, thus providing indirect support to First Aid for Depression. Moreover, directed imagery training can be extended to induce positive mood and develop antidepressive pathways (see Chapter 11).

## A FRESH APPROACH TO TREATMENT

Because the First Aid technique can ameliorate symptoms of depression quite dramatically, under certain circumstances I have used the technique in the first session, before taking a detailed history. A brief history should always be taken, to assess for suicidal ideation. If the therapist is convinced that no suicidal ideation exists, the First Aid technique can be used in the following situations:

- The patient is referred by a psychiatrist or other mental health professional, and a full report detailing the history and symptoms of depression is provided.
- The patient has chronic depression, and the recent episode is exacerbated by psychosocial factors.

- The patient is not currently suicidal, and he does not plan to carry out suicide.
- The patient is not presenting severe psychomotor retardation, and no serious vegetative symptoms are present.
- The patient is known to the therapist.

If the therapist is satisfied that the history taken is sufficient, it is not productive for either the patient or therapist to repeat a detailed history. This may take up an entire long session in itself. The patient may be denied treatment until the next session, which, depending on the therapist's schedule, may not be for another week or later. Such an approach, although inevitable at times, may frustrate and distress the patient, especially in the case of a chronically depressed person, who may have seen many clinicians and therapists in the past and endured a similar routine. Very often such a process puts the patient off to the extent that they do not return for treatment, and the cycle of failure to resolve symptoms continues.

## SUMMARY

First Aid for depression is ideal for acute situational depression. Some empirical evidence suggests that a brief intervention such as directed imagery can reduce both self-rated and behavioral indices of depression, thus providing indirect support for the First Aid technique for depression. Although the initial improvement in depressive level gradually diminishes over time, the technique provides evidence to the patient (especially to someone with a chronically depressive affect) that the depressive cycle can be broken. This gives the patient hope that the depression can be alleviated: The treatment is seen as positive, and the therapeutic relationship is strengthened.

## REFERENCES

Alladin, A. (1989). Cognitive hypnotherapy for depression. In D. Waxman, D. Pederson, I. Wilkie, & P. Mellett (Eds.), *Hypnosis: The 4th European Congress at Oxford* (pp. 175–182). London: Whurr Publishers.

Alladin, A. (1992). Hypnosis with depression. *American Journal of Preventive Psychiatry and Neurology*, 3(3), 13–18.

Alladin, A. (1992a). Depression as a dissociative state. *Hypnos: Swedish Journal of Hypnosis in Psychotherapy and Psychosomatic Medicine*, 19, 243–253.

Alladin, A. (1994). Cognitive hypnotherapy with depression. *Journal of Cognitive Psychotherapy: An International Quarterly*, 8(4), 275–288.

Alladin, A. (2006). Cognitive hypnotherapy for treating depression. In R. Chapman (Ed.) *The clinical use of hypnosis in cognitive behavior therapy: A practitioner's casebook* (pp. 139–187). New York: Springer Publishing Company.

Alladin, A., & Heap, M. (1991). Hypnosis and depression. In M. Heap & W. Dryden (Eds.), *Hypnotherapy: A handbook*, (pp. 49–67). Open University Press.

Burtle, V. (1975). Learning in the appositional mind: Imagery in the treatment of depression. *Dissertation Abstract International*, 36(II–B), 5781. Los Angeles: California School of Professional Psychology.

Gold, S.R., Jarvinen, P.J., & Teague, R.G. (1982). Imagery elaboration and clarity in modifying college students' depression. *Journal of Clinical Psychology*, 38, 312–314.

Jarvinen, P.J., & Gold, S.R. (1981). Imagery as an aid in reducing depression. *Journal of Clinical Psychology*, 37(3), 523–529.

Lipsky, M.J., Kassinove, H., & Miller, N.J. (1980). Effects of rational-emotive therapy, rational role reversal, and rational-emotive imagery on the emotional adjustment of community mental health centre patients. *Journal of Consulting and Clinical Psychology*, 48(3), 366–374.

Overlade, D.C. (1986). First aid for depression. In E.T. Dowd & J.M. Healy (Eds.), *Case studies in hypnotherapy* (pp. 23–33). New York: Guilford Press.

Reardon, J.P., & Tossi, D.J. (1977). The effects of rational stage directed imagery on self-concept and reduction of psychological stress in adolescent delinquent females. *Journal of Clinical Psychology*, 33, 1084–1092.

Schultz, K.D. (1978). Imagery and the control of depression. In J.L. Singer & K.S. Pope (Eds.), *The power of human imagination: New methods in psychotherapy* (pp. 281–307). New York: Plenum Press.

Schultz, K.D. (1984). The use of imagery in alleviating depression. In A.A. Sheik (Ed.), *Imagination and healing* (pp. 129–158). New York: Baywood.

Schultz, K.D. (2003). The use of imagery in alleviating depression. In A.A. Sheikh (Ed.), *Healing images: The role of imagination in health* (pp. 343–380). New York: Baywood.

Sheikh, A.A. (Ed.) (2003). *Healing images: The role of imagination in health*. New York: Baywood.

Sirota, A.D., & Schwartz, G.E. (1982). Facial muscle patterning and lateralization during elation and depression imagery. *Journal of Abnormal Psychology*, 91(1), 25–34.

Velton, E. (1968). A laboratory task for induction of mood states. *Behavior Research and Therapy*, 6, 473–482.

# Cognitive Behavior Therapy

Chapter 2 reviewed the cognitive model of depression, which states that depression is often maintained and exacerbated by exaggerated or biased ways of thinking. Cognitive behavior therapy (CBT) is utilized to help depressed patients recognize and modify their idiosyncratic style of thinking through the application of evidence and logic. CBT uses some very well-known and tested reason-based models such as the Socratic logic-based dialogues and Aristotle's method of collecting and categorizing information about the world (Leahy, 2003). CBT therapists engage their patients in scientific and rational thinking by guiding them to examine the presupposition, validity, and meaning of their beliefs that lead to their depressive affect. Because CBT techniques are fully described in several excellent books (e.g., Beck, 1995), they are not described in detail here. Within the cognitive-hypnosis (CH) framework, I adopt (Alladin, 2006, 2006a) the following sequential progression of CBT, which can be extended over four to six sessions. However, the number of CBT sessions is determined by the needs of the patient and the severity of the presenting symptoms:

- Explanation of the cognitive model of depression
- Reading assignment (to read first three chapters from *Feeling Good: The New Mood Therapy* [Burns, 1999])
- Patient identification of cognitive distortions ruminated on
- Patient logging of dysfunctional thoughts on the CAB Form
- Introduction of disputation or restructuring of cognitive distortions
- Introduction of the ABCDE Form
- Identification and restructuring of core beliefs
- Development of the habit of monitoring and restructuring negative beliefs

The progression of CBT is illustrated by describing the first two CBT sessions carried out with Patty, whose case was formulated in Chapter 7.

## FIRST SESSION

### Explanation of Cognitive Model of Depression

In the first CBT session, the patient is provided a detailed but practical explanation of the cognitive model of depression. This psychoeducational session usually lasts about an hour. Some beginning therapists may think it is a waste of time to spend so much time in psychoeducation. However, Ledley, Marx, and Heimberg (2005) have listed several advantages for spending one or two sessions in explaining the CBT model to the patient:

- It provides a nonthreatening means of interaction.
- It helps to establish and strengthen rapport.
- It is a learning process for patient and therapist.
- It actively involves both patient and therapist.
- It facilitates ongoing case conceptualization.
- It provides open discussion and collaboration between patient and therapist.
- It provides a context within which the therapist may normalize patient experiences.
- It allows opportunity to discuss how problems are interfering with patient's functioning.
- The whole process helps the patient gain confidence in the treatment.

It is important for the therapist not to deliver the psychoeducational material in a lecture format. Such an approach will damage therapeutic rapport. It is important for the therapist to strike a balance between sharing information and keeping the patient involved. The excerpt from Patty's first CBT session illustrates this balance in the presentation of the psychoeducational material covered.

### ABC Model of Psychopathology

The patient is given a practical explanation for understanding the cognitive model of psychopathology, specifically the cognitive model of depression. While explaining the model, the therapist writes the salient points on a piece of paper or on a board. Writing provides a visual representation of the model, and both the patient and therapist can refer to the notes to check on a point.

### Redefining Depression

*Therapist:* At the end of our last session, we concluded that you have a major depressive disorder. Although this term is a useful description, it's not very meaningful to you in terms of your experience. I am going to redefine your condition. Your condition can be described as an emotional problem or an emotional disorder, and we refer to it as an emotional disorder when it gets severe. An emotional disorder has two main characteristics. First, a person with an emotional disorder has excessive negative feelings. This means the person has lots of negative feelings that the person does not want, but can't get rid of, even when the person is in a situation where the person should be having a good time. Do you feel this way?

*Patty:* Yes, most of the time.

*Therapist:* Secondly, a person with an emotional disorder tends to overreact to situations. That is, the feeling is out of proportion to the situation. Do you feel this way?

*Patty:* Yes.

*Therapist:* In this session, I am going to explain to you why you have excessive negative feeling and why you overreact to situations. If you know the reasons why, then you may be able to do something about it.

*Patty:* I would really be interested to know why.

### Explanations about Emotions

*Therapist:* Since we are focusing on emotions, let's talk about emotions for a while. The English language is very rich in describing emotions. There are over 300 adjectives used to describe emotions or feelings. But they can be categorized either as positive or negative emotions. In our discussion, we are going to use words like emotions, feelings, and reactions interchangeably. That is, they mean the same thing. We say we are emotional when we are reacting or expressing a feeling. Can you give me some examples of positive feelings?

*Patty:* Happy, confident, feeling good.

*Therapist:* That's right. And also sense of success, sense of achievement, joy, and so on. Now can you give me some examples of negative feelings?

*Patty:* Sad, angry, anxious.

*Therapist:* That's right. Other negative feelings are guilt, fear, feeling depressed, and so on. OK, we have both negative and positive feelings, but from where do they come? Are we born with feelings, or do we learn them?

*Patty:* We are born with feelings.

*Therapist:* It seems this way, but we are not really born with feelings and emotions. We learn them.

*Patty:* But how come a baby cries?

*Therapist:* When a baby is born, it experiences distress and gratification. If the baby is hungry or wet, it is distressed and cries. But if the baby is warm and fed, it is gratified and usually goes to sleep. In other words, the baby has the ability to feel feelings and emotions, but a newborn baby does not know when or where to express feelings. The baby has to learn how, when, and where to express feelings, because most feelings are related to people or situations.

*Patty:* I did not realize this. I did not know that feelings are learned. Now that you mentioned it, it makes sense.

*Therapist:* There are three lines of evidence to prove that emotions are learned. First, as we discovered, a newborn baby does know what feelings to express in different situations. Second, different people feel different feelings in the same situations. Third, different cultures express different feelings in the same situation. For example, in some cultures, people are grieved at a funeral. In other cultures, they celebrate at a funnel. For example, in certain parts of Ireland and Scotland, they have a wake when someone dies.

*Patty:* I find this very interesting.

*Therapist:* The reason why we are attaching so much importance to learning is because, if emotions are learned, then we can change them or modify them.

### The Link between Emotion and Cognition

In this part of the psychoeducation, the therapist helps the patient understand the link between emotion and cognition.

*Therapist:* Now, we know that emotions and feelings are learned, but what triggers them? We don't laugh or cry for no apparent reasons. What triggers feelings?

*Patty:* People. Something happens.

*Therapist:* That's right. When something happens. This is what we call an *event* or a *situation*. There is a relationship here. When a positive event or situation occurs, we have a positive feeling. But when a negative event or situation occurs, we have a negative feeling. For example, suppose a person close to you wins a million dollars. How would you feel?

*Patty:* I would feel happy for the person.

*Therapist:* But let's suppose your close friend is involved in a serious accident and is in the hospital. How would you feel?

*Patty:* I would feel sad and distressed.

*Therapist:* But these are current situations, things happening now. Events can also be past or future. For example, if you think of a good event that occurred many years ago, you will feel good about it because it was a happy event.

*Patty:* I understand this, but what do you mean by an event being in the future?

*Therapist:* Let's suppose you are having this therapy with me, and you believe that in 6 months you will improve, as the literature predicts. You will feel happy, although you are not there yet. So the past, the present, or the future can influence us now.

*Patty:* Is that why some people get upset when you mention something about the past or about the future?

*Therapist:* That's right. You seem to be very perceptive, Patty!

*Patty:* I find this interesting. I have always enjoyed psychology.

*Therapist:* I am glad you find this meaningful. Let's summarize what we have covered so far. We discovered that events or situations trigger our feelings, that is, events or situations, depending on whether they are negative or positive, determine our feelings. In other words, we are saying that events cause us to feel happy or sad. In other words, events are responsible for how we feel. We are not responsible for how we feel. Events are responsible.

*Patty:* That's right.

*Therapist:* Let's examine whether events and situations are responsible for how we feel, and that we are not responsible for how we feel.

*Patty:* OK.

*Therapist:* Let's take divorce as an example. Imagine 100 people got divorced this morning. These 100 people represent a representative sample of our society. They are from all walks of life. How do you think they felt after they got their divorces?

*Patty:* I suppose some felt relieved and some felt distressed.

*Therapist:* Would you like to speculate on what percent felt relieved or happy and what percent felt unhappy or distressed?

*Patty:* I would say 70% felt depressed and 30% felt relieved.

*Therapist:* Now, if there were 100 people in this room and we ask them the same question, people would give different answers. Some may say, like you, 70% will feel depressed while 30% will feel happy. Others may say 50–50 or 60–40 or 80–20. But I bet you no one will say 100% will feel happy or sad.

*Patty:* I agree with you.

*Therapist:* If this is true, then we are contradicting ourselves. Earlier on we agreed that (pointing to the notes) events or situations are responsible for how we feel, and we are not responsible for how we feel. If this were true, then everyone will feel either happy or depressed since it's the same situation for everyone—that is, everyone got divorced.

*Patty:* Well, different people have different reactions.

*Therapist:* True. Reactions are feelings or emotions. If the event was responsible for how we feel then everyone will feel the same, since it's the same situation.

*Patty:* I see what you mean. You mean it's not the event that causes the feeling.

*Therapist:* You're right. The event can't be causing the feeling, otherwise everyone who got divorced would have felt either sad or happy. We agreed that some were feeling sad and others were feeling happy. This would prove that the event is not responsible for how we feel. Patty, if the event is not responsible, what do you think is responsible for how we feel?

*Patty:* Our brain.

*Therapist:* It may be coming from our brain, but can you be more specific?

*Patty:* Our experience.

*Therapist:* You are moving in the right direction. Can you be a bit more specific?

*Patty:* What we remember from our experience.

*Therapist:* You're right. It's not the event that causes us to feel sad or happy, but it's our perception of the event. The way we evaluate or appraise the event, based on our experience and learning, determines how we feel. The event simply acts as a trigger. I am sure you already knew that but never thought about it systematically the way we are analyzing it.

*Patty:* You're right. I always knew that my thinking is too negative.

*Therapist:* The mental process that's involved in thinking, evaluation, self-talk, and inner dialogue is called *cognition*. So it's our cognition that determines how we feel and not the situation on its own. Let's examine the example about divorce a bit further. What types of cognition do you think went into the person's head who felt happy after divorce?

*Patty:* I am free. I can marry the person I really love.

*Therapist:* And what kind of cognition in the person who felt sad after the divorce was granted?

*Patty:* I am a failure, I failed again. I will be lonely.

*Therapist:* Because cognitions determine how we feel, cognitions can be tragic. I am sure you have come across a person who is doing the wrong things, but the person believes he or she is doing the right thing. And the person will tell you "I know I'm right because I believe it." Believing in something does not make you right, because we are not born with beliefs. We learn them, and it's possible for us to learn the wrong beliefs based on our experience. Or the person may say "I'm right because I feel it." Feeling does not make you right, because feelings are created by our thinking. The thinking may be wrong. Have you come across such people?

*Patty:* Sure. My friend Jennifer is just like that.

*Therapist:* It's tragic for two reasons. First, the person continues to believe in something that's not helpful, although it continues to cause lots of difficulties in the person's life. And second, the person is not even aware that the belief is creating the problems.

*Patty:* I always knew that my thinking was causing my depression, but how do I change it?

*Therapist:* The main purpose of cognitive behavior therapy or CBT is to show you how to restructure your thinking.

*Patty:* But how can you change it when I have been thinking this way all my life?

*Therapist:* It's not easy, but it can be changed. That's why we were attaching so much importance to learning. Since your thinking is learned, it can be changed or modified. CBT shows you how to do this.

*Patty:* I am impatient. I want to know more about this.

*Therapist:* I am glad you find this interesting. Let's talk a bit more about cognitions, and then we will address how you start working with your thinking. We mentioned that cognitions can be tragic. Let's examine this a bit further. In other words, cognitions can be accurate, helpful, adaptive, and rational or they can be inaccurate, unhelpful, unadaptive, and irrational, and we don't know about it. We simply believe what we believe in, and our thinking becomes automatic, never questioning or paying attention to our beliefs. Our beliefs are learned and shaped by our experience. David Burns in his book, *Feeling Good: The New Mood Therapy*, talks about 10 kinds of cognitive distortions. Cognitive distortions are automatic negative thoughts that produce bad or negative feelings. So, whenever an event occurs, we immediately think negatively or maladaptively. There is a relationship between how we think and how we feel. If an event occurs, and you think adaptively about it, you have a balanced or an adaptive feeling. But if your thinking is distorted, then you feel upset about it. Let's illustrate this by an example. But before I go on, let's check your take on this.

*Patty:* Everything you say makes sense. You mentioned the book by David Burns. Should I read the book?

*Therapist:* Yes. Reading the book, certain chapters at a time, will be part of the homework that we will be talking about later on. First, let's talk about the example. Imagine the case of Mary who is a 45-year-old married woman with migraine headaches. Mary has been suffering from migraines for over 10 years, but her headaches have become very frequent and severe lately. She used to have two migraines per month and lately she has been having one or two migraines per week. So Mary went to see her family physician, who got concerned and referred Mary to a neurologist for a full check up to rule out any organic cause for her migraines. A month ago, the results of the tests came out, and they were all negative. Mary's physician reassured her that there is nothing physically wrong with her, but he believes the severity and frequency of her migraines have increased due to stress. Mary has been under lots of stress in the past few months. Her mother, who has a terminal illness, has been living with Mary and her family. Very often Mary had to stay up all night to nurse her mother. The doctor advised her to continue to take her medication and reassured her that her headaches will improve once the stress is resolved.

Two weeks ago, Mary saw a program on television about a holistic treatment program for migraine. This is a 4-month out-patient program consisting of meditation, hypnotherapy, stress management, selective medication, and clinical biofeedback. The TV program was an hour long, and it consisted of different individuals giving their testimonials about the treatment. Some had migraines for over 10 years, and 85% of the people who participated in the program significantly improved. Before the end of the TV program, the commentator indicated that one should see one's family physician first before joining the treatment program, because migraine can be due to various medical conditions or a brain tumor. At the end of the program, Mary became convinced that she had a brain tumor and she started panicking and became very depressed. Why do you think Mary started panicking and became depressed?

*Patty:* Because she thought she had brain tumor.

*Therapist:* Why is that belief irrational—that is, not based on facts?

*Patty:* It's irrational for Mary to believe she has a brain tumor because she does not have one.

*Therapist:* How do we know this? What are the facts?

*Patty:* Because she saw a neurologist, and all the tests were negative.

*Therapist:* Now let's suppose Mary looks at the information accurately. She says to herself that she is glad there is nothing organically wrong with her and, therefore, this new treatment program gives her hope. She would like to ask her doctor to refer her to this program. In this case, how would Mary feel?

*Patty:* Relieved and hopeful.

*Therapist:* In this case, she is not depressed but not cured either. But her feeling is balanced, realistic, or adaptive. This example clearly illustrates how thinking determines our feelings. The reason why I am telling you all this is because I want to show you how to change your cognitive distortions. From our interview last week, we identified several cognitive distortions that appear to be maintaining your depression, and often they exacerbate your symptoms. This is why we decided to give you a course of CBT.

*Patty:* My psychiatrist also believes I need CBT.

*Therapist:* I am glad you and your psychiatrist agree with the treatment. But before we start CBT, it is recommended that patients learn to identify their automatic negative cognitions first. To achieve this, I am going to suggest some homework for you.

### Homework

For homework, the patient is advised to read the first three chapters from *Feeling Good: The New Mood Therapy* (Burns, 1999) and to log the CAB Form (Table 8.1). By logging the CAB Form, patients are able to identify their cognitive distortions and monitor their negative feelings. This exercise helps them understand the relationship between their automatic thoughts and their feelings.

### Bibliotherapy

*Therapist:* To start with, I would like you to read the first three chapters from the *Feeling Good* book. First read chapters 1 and 2, and then read chapter 3 a couple of times. I would like you to become familiar with the 10 types of cognitive distortions that Burns describes, and identify how many of these distortions apply to you. Make a note of it.

*Patty:* I have the book. My psychiatrist recommended it, but I have never read it.

*Therapist:* I am glad you have the book, but just focus on the first three chapters for now.

### Logging the CAB Form

*Therapist:* The second part of the homework involves logging the CAB Form (the patient is handed a CAB Form). From now on, whenever you feel upset, anxious, or depressed, write your feelings down in column C, just as this patient has recorded his (pointing to column C on the CAB Form). Then rate how much of these feelings you feel; "0" representing very low intensity and "100" representing the worst you can feel. This is purely subjective. It's your own personal rating of how bad you feel.

*Patty:* When do I fill in this form?

*Therapist:* Whenever you experience a negative feeling. Of course, you may not be able to do it when you are with other people or when you are doing something. Try to do it as soon as it's convenient for you to write down your negative feelings. Then write down the situation that triggered these feelings in column A (pointing to column A on the CAB Form). Then identify the thoughts that went through your mind, just as this patient has recorded his (pointing to the example listed in column B) and rate how much you believe in these thoughts on a scale of "0" to "100"; "0" indicating you have very little belief in your thought and "100" indicating you completely believe in your thought. Does this sound OK to you?

*Patty:* How often do I fill in the form?

**Table 8.1.  CAB form for monitoring irrational beliefs/thoughts/images/daydreams related to events/situations**

| Date C = Emotions | A = Facts or Events | B = Automatic Thoughts About A |
|---|---|---|
| 1. Specify sad/ anxious/angry, etc. 2. Rate degree of emotion 0–100 | Describe: 1. Actual event that activated unpleasant emotion/reaction 2. Images, daydreams, recollection leading to unpleasant emotion | 1. Write automatic thoughts that preceded emotions/reactions 2. Rate belief in automatic thoughts 0–100% |
| *Sept. 06/02* | | |
| *Depressed (75)* *Unhappy (100)* *Miserable (90)* | *Thinking of going to grandson's Christening party tomorrow* | *I won't enjoy it (100)* *I can't cope with it (100)* *Everyone will hate me (90)* *I will spoil it for everyone (90)* *I can never be happy again (100)* |

*Therapist:* Complete three of these forms (handing three blank forms to Patty). By completing these forms, you will begin to see the link between B and C. Most people pay attention to either their thoughts or the events, very rarely paying attention to their thinking. Since we are going to work with your thinking, it's important for us to identify your automatic thoughts. Because you have been thinking in this way for such a long time, your thinking has becoming automatic, so you may not be even be aware of your thinking. From now on, I would like you to have a "third inner ear," listening to your thoughts whenever you get upset. Bring the completed forms with you to your next session. In the next session, we will be focusing on restructuring your thinking, so we would need some examples from your homework, so that I can show you how to change your negative thinking.

## SECOND SESSION

### Restructuring of Cognitive Distortions

During the second session of CBT, patients are introduced to disputation (D) after they have had the opportunity to log the CAB Form for a week. The homework provides patients with the opportunity to identify and categorize their negative thoughts and to examine how these thoughts are related to their depression. This preparatory work sets the stage for evaluating and challenging their negative thoughts. A variety of techniques for testing the validity of negative thoughts are described, but it should be borne in mind that some negative thoughts may be true. It should be remembered that CBT does not advocate the "power of positive thinking," but rather the "power of identifying whatever is being thought" (Leahy, 2003). CBT takes a constructivist approach to therapy by recognizing that an individual's construction and interpretation of reality are based on unique information, personal categories, and biases in perception or cognition.

Disputation forms part of the Cognitive Restructuring Form (Table 8.2). This form is an expanded version of the CAB Form; it includes two more columns (D = Disputation; E = Consequences of Disputation). To get a better grasp on how to complete this form, patients are given a completed version of the Cognitive Restructuring Form (Table 8.3) (with disputation of cognitive distortions in column D and the modification of emotional and behavioral responses in column E as a consequence of cognitive disputation).

### *Agenda Setting*

Agenda setting is generally considered to be essential in CBT, although the structure of the session may vary. According to Sanders and Wills (2005), agenda setting maximizes the use of time in a therapy session, ensures certain items are covered, and aids the patient's memory of the session. Ledley, Marx, and Heimberg (2005) have identified seven components forming the basic framework of a generic CBT session. These include:

- Review with the patient about the week.
- Collaboratively set the session agenda.
- Review the homework.
- Conduct the main session content based on treatment plan.
- Assign new homework (based on main session content).

**Table 8.2.** Cognitive restructuring form

| Date | A Activating Event | B Irrational Beliefs | C Consequences | D Disputation | E Effect of Disputation |
|---|---|---|---|---|---|
| | Describe actual event, stream of thoughts, daydream, etc. leading to unpleasant feelings. | Write automatic thoughts and images that came in your mind. Rate beliefs or images 0–100% | 1. <u>Emotion</u>: specify sad, anxious or angry. Rate feelings 1–100% <br> 2. <u>Physiological</u>: Palpitations, pain, dizzy, sweat, etc. <br> 3. <u>Behavioral</u>: Avoidance, in bed. <br> 4. <u>Conclusion</u>: Reaching conclusions, self-affirmation. | Challenge the automatic thoughts and images. Rate belief in rational response/image 0–100% | 1. <u>Emotion</u>: Re-rate your emotion 1–100% <br> 2. <u>Physiological</u>: Changes in bodily reactions (i.e. less shaking, less tense, etc.) <br> 3. <u>Behavioral</u>: Action taken after disputation. <br> 4. <u>Conclusion</u>: Reappraise your conclusion and initial decision. Future beliefs in similar situation. |

**Table 8.3.   Completed cognitive restructuring form**

| Date | A<br>Activating<br>Event | B<br>Irrational<br>Beliefs | C<br>Consequences | D<br>Disputation | E<br>Effect of<br>Disputation |
|---|---|---|---|---|---|
| | Describe actual event, stream of thoughts, daydream, etc. leading to unpleasant feelings. | Write automatic thoughts and images that came in your mind. Rate beliefs or images 0–100% | 1. Emotion: specify sad, anxious or angry. Rate feelings 1–100%<br>2. Physiological: Palpitations, pain, dizzy, sweat, etc.<br>3. Behavioral: Avoidance, in bed.<br>4. Conclusion: Reaching conclusions, self-affirmation. | Challenge the automatic thoughts and images. Rate belief in rational response/image 0–100% | 1. Emotion: Re-rate your emotion 1–100%<br>2. Physiological: Changes in bodily reactions (i.e., less shaking, less tense, etc.)<br>3. Behavioral: Action taken after disputation.<br>4. Conclusion: Reappraise your conclusion and initial decision. Future beliefs in similar situation. |

| 05/20/2005 | A worked example: Thinking of going to grandson's Christening party | 1. I won't enjoy it (100) 2. I can't cope with it (90) 3. Everyone will hate me (90) 4. I will spoil it for everyone (100) 5. I can never be happy so what's the point of going (100) | 1. Depressed (75), unhappy (100), miserable (90) 2. Weak, tired, head heavy 3. Don't want to go, prefer staying in bed 4. I will never be able to enjoy myself again | 1. How do I know I won't enjoy it? The chances are I may like it being in company (60) 2. I may still feel depressed, but I can cope with it. Nothing bad will happen (80) 3. No one hates you when you feel down, it's just my wrong belief (80) 4. I may be quiet but not spoil it for all (90) 5. I've felt this way in the past, but have always recovered/come on top (100) | 1. Less depressed (20), not too unhappy (30), no longer feeling miserable (0) 2. Still feeling tired and weak but head feels light, and feels like making a move 3. Out of bed, ironing clothes for the party tomorrow, wish to be present at party 4. Even if I feel depressed, I can make myself happy by going out to social functions |

- Summarize the session by asking the patient what she learned in the session.
- Check with the patient about any questions, concerns, or issues.

The therapist should have a rough agenda in mind before going into each session, although it is essential to involve the patient in planning the session. The main therapy contents are covered between reviewing the completed homework and assigning new homework.

### Review of the Week

*Therapist:* Patty, how have you been since our last meeting?

*Patty:* Still depressed, but I feel hopeful.

*Therapist:* How bad was your depression?

*Patty:* Not as bad as a few weeks ago. At least I did not feel hopeless.

*Therapist:* To what do you attribute your hopefulness?

*Patty:* The last two sessions with you. You seem to understand how I feel. And the readings have helped.

### Review of Homework

*Therapist:* Did you get an opportunity to read the three chapters?

*Patty:* I read the first two chapters once as you suggested, but read chapter 3 three times. I was surprised that most of the cognitive distortions apply to me.

*Therapist:* Are you convinced that negative cognitions create bad feelings?

*Patty:* I guess I always knew that, but never thought about it the way you explained. The last session made it easier for me to understand the book. I hate to think that I have been making myself depressed by dwelling on all those negative thoughts.

*Therapist:* I am glad you see the connection between your cognitive distortions and your depression. However, I would like to reassure you that it's not your fault. You were not thinking negatively because you wanted to, but your mind, based on your experience, was programmed to think that way. Now that you know that your thinking, to a large extent, determines and maintains your depression, we can help you learn to think differently. How did you find your homework with recording your thoughts?

*Patty:* I found it easy to record my thinking since I have so many negative thoughts going in my mind. The example helped a lot. I felt embarrassed to write down some of the thoughts because they are so stupid.

*Therapist:* Can I have a look at your forms? (Patty hands the three completed forms to the therapist.) I see you did a very good job. You should not feel embarrassed to write down your thoughts, however insensible they may appear. I am not going to judge you because of your thinking. I am familiar with the thoughts that go through depressed people's minds. Moreover, writing them down makes you realize how irrational some of the thoughts are and in turn encourages you to give them up. Now I am going to show you how to do the disputation, and then we will talk about further homework.

### Cognitive Restructuring

*Therapist:* This week we are introducing you to a new form, the Cognitive Restructuring Form. This form is an expanded version of the CAB Form (handing a blank and a completed Cognitive Restructuring Form to Patty), with two extra columns D and E. In column D, we do the disputation, and in column E we record the effects of the disputation, as you can see in this completed Cognitive Restructuring Form. You also notice that this form goes from A to E. In the CAB Form, we assigned C to the first column, because people are more aware of their feelings. But now that you have experience recording the form for a week, you can record on either column A or C first. In the Cognitive Restructuring Form, we start with A and moves on to E because it forms an alphabetical sequence. You also notice we have broken C into four categories: 1, representing emotions or feelings, as in the CAB Form; 2, representing physical or physiological changes; 3, representing behavior; and 4, representing conclusion or self-affirmation.

What this means is that any experience has four components. When we experience an emotion, we often produce physiological changes that affect our behavior, and then we reach a conclusion about our experience. For example, in this Completed Cognitive Restructuring Form (pointing to the form), the patient is feeling unhappy, depressed, and miserable, which make her feel weak and tired, and her head feels heavy. As a consequence, her behavior is affected; she prefers staying in bed. From this emotional, physical, and behavioral experience, she concludes that she will never be able to enjoy herself, and this reinforces or confirms her underlying belief that she will never be able to feel good. Do you follow?

*Patty:* You mean, because a person feels bad, the person concludes that he or she will always feels bad?

*Therapist:* Precisely. Such conclusions act as a form of posthypnotic suggestions, which we will discuss when we do hypnosis in future sessions.

*Patty:* That's me. I'm always telling myself that I will never amount to anything.

*Therapist:* We will be working with these beliefs in our CBT sessions. Now let me show you how to do the disputation. We take each statement in turn from column B and examine its validity. The first statement says "I won't enjoy it," and she believes it 100%. What kind of a cognitive distortion is this?

*Patty:* Fortune Teller Error and Overgeneralization.

*Therapist:* You're right, Patty. It shows you studied chapter 3 carefully. But it's also All-or-Nothing Thinking. Do you agree?

*Patty:* Yes, because there are different levels of enjoyment.

*Therapist:* Yes, you're right again. Enjoyment can be placed on a continuum (therapist draws on a piece of paper); it's not either we enjoy or don't enjoy; we can have different degrees of enjoyment. The way to dispute this statement is something like this: "How do

I know I won't enjoy? I have not been there yet, so how do I know. It's true that in the past I went to some places I did not like. But I also remember many times I did not want to go to a function, but once I got there, I had fun. So forcing myself to go my grandson's christening party might help me get out of my depression, and it will give me an opportunity to see other people whom I have not seen for a while. Moreover, it's important for me to be at my grandson's christening party. Even if I don't enjoy myself fully, it does not matter." Because of lack of space, the patient has written a shortened version of it in column D. Does this give you a flavor of how we dispute?

*Patty:* So you don't just think positive, you try to reason with your wrong beliefs.

*Therapist:* That's right. First, we recognize that the belief is irrational, then we try to categorize it according to David Burns' list of cognitive distortions. For CBT to be effective, it's important to question and challenge the beliefs underlying the cognitions. Let's examine the second statement: "I can't cope with it." What kind a cognitive distortion is this statement?

*Patty:* Fortune Teller Error, Overgeneralization, and All-or-Nothing Thinking.

*Therapist:* You're right. This is how we dispute this belief. "I have not gone to the party yet, so how do I know I can't cope with it? Somehow, I am coping with my depression. Going to the party is not that demanding. Nothing bad will happen to me. Somehow I will cope. Coping is not either you cope or don't cope. I don't have to be able to cope 100% to go somewhere."

*Patty:* That's me. Whenever I have to do something, I always think I can't cope with it, and this saps my confidence, and then I refrain from doing anything.

*Therapist:* This is what we call *catastrophizing*. Anxious or depressed individuals catastrophize. They anticipate the worst. But once they are in the situation, their feelings are not as bad as they anticipated. In column D, the patient has written a summary of her disputation. Now let's work with the third statement from column B, which says: "Everyone will hate me." What kind of a thinking error is this?

*Patty:* All-or-Nothing Thinking, Magnification, and Fortune Teller Error.

*Therapist:* That's right. The best way to dispute this belief is to use the *double standard technique*. This technique relates to the fact that anxious or depressed individuals sympathize with people who have anxiety or depression, but they believe other people will be unsympathetic to them because they are anxious or depressed.

*Patty:* I always do that.

*Therapist:* Let me show you how you dispute this. Imagine you go to a party, and you come across a friend who looks nervous or depressed. Would you hate the person?

*Patty:* No.

*Therapist:* Would you say "Go away. You don't have the right to be here because you are anxious, depressed?"

*Patty:* No. On the contrary, I will reassure the person and make the person feel comfortable.

*Therapist:* Then why should others hate you if you feel anxious or depressed?

*Patty:* I see your point. But what if someone hates you?

*Therapist:* The way to deal with that is to have a realistic view of the world. Whoever you are, however popular you are, someone is going to dislike you. Let's take the example of Abraham Lincoln and Mahatma Gandhi. Abraham Lincoln was such a kind person, but guess what? Someone shot him. Mahatma Gandhi was such a simple man and, through peaceful means, he liberated India from the mighty British Empire—and guess what? Someone shot him. Now you can imagine, we are ordinary people; someone is likely to hate us. But also many people in the world like us. If the majority of the people like you and a minority hates you, can you live with it?

*Patty:* I never thought about it this way. I prefer to focus on the majority's view.

*Therapist:* You can notice in column D the patient, after disputation, now believes with 80% of certainty that people don't hate you when you feel down. Rating the new beliefs gives you a sense of your success with your disputation. The higher the rating, the greater will be your belief in your new way of thinking. Now let's focus on the fourth statement from the list, which says: "I will spoil it for everyone." Apart from the cognitive distortions we have already mentioned, what kind a cognitive distortion is this belief?

*Patty:* I am not sure.

*Therapist:* I will give you a clue: It's the last on the list and starts with "p."

*Patty:* Personalization.

*Therapist:* Right. She is attributing responsibility to herself. If anything goes wrong, she will blame herself for it. How do you dispute this one?

*Patty:* Well, being depressed does not mean you make everyone depressed. Your depression has no relationship to the party. Some people may not even notice you are depressed.

*Therapist:* Right. When you are at a party, people form little cliques of four or five people each. Let's suppose there are 50 people at the party, and you belong to one of these cliques. Because you are depressed, you may be quiet or a bit withdrawn, but you don't spoil it for everyone.

*Patty:* How silly. I always think it's my fault when anything goes wrong.

*Therapist:* If this thought occurs in your mind next time, do you know how to dispute it?

*Patty:* Yes.

*Therapist:* Now, let's examine the effects of disputation in column E. Since B causes C, disputation of B is likely to change C, and this is what we notice in column E.

*Homework*

*Therapist:* I am going to give you some blank forms (hands three Cognitive Restructuring Forms to Patty) and, from now on, whenever you feel upset or depressed, complete columns A, B, and C. Then dispute the beliefs listed in column D, then record the effects of disputation in column E. Also be sure to rate your feelings in columns C and E, and your beliefs in columns B and D. Study the Completed Cognitive Restructuring Form; it provides a model for your homework. Does this sound OK to you?

*Patty:* I find the session very useful, and I am really looking forward to do this.

*Therapist:* I am so happy to see you so motivated. I would also like you to read chapters 4 and 5. Is this OK?

*Patty:* Yes.

*Therapist:* How was the session for you, and what did you learn from this session?

*Patty:* I find the CBT very helpful. Now I know what I was doing wrong, and now I know what to do to fight my depression. I am already beginning to feel better, and I feel hopeful.

**OTHER CBT TECHNIQUES**

The rest of the CBT sessions are conducted in a format similar to Session Two and, as the need arises based on the case formulation, other techniques are introduced. The techniques may include behavioral strategies (described in Chapter 13), imagery training (discussed in Chapters 9 and 11), and identification of core beliefs (described in Chapter 10). Part of each session should also be devoted to reducing helplessness, hopelessness, and suicidal behaviors. Chapters 11 and 12 address these issues. It is also important for the therapist to continue to socialize the patient into CBT and the cognitive model of depression throughout the course of therapy. This approach directs the patients to pay close attention to her negative cognitive rumination and encourages her to restructure her negative cognitions until it becomes a habit. Gradually, she becomes socialized into the circular feedback model of depression (CFMD) and becomes aware of the multiple factors that trigger and maintain her depressive affect. Moreover, she learns various strategies to deal with depression.

**SUMMARY**

This chapter provided a practical demonstration of how to introduce CBT to the patient and how to start restructuring cognitive distortions. Later chapters describe various cognitive and noncognitive strategies that can be easily integrated with CBT. It is important for the therapist to continue to socialize the patient into the CFMD throughout the whole course of therapy.

**REFERENCES**

Alladin, A. (2006). Cognitive hypnotherapy for treating depression. In R. Chapman (Ed.), *The clinical use of hypnosis in cognitive behavior therapy: A practitioner's casebook* (pp. 139–187). New York: Springer Publishing Company.
Alladin, A. (2006a). Experiential cognitive hypnotherapy: Strate-

gies for relapse prevention in depression. In M. Yapko (Ed.), *Hypnosis and treating depression: Advances in clinical practice* (pp. 281–313). New York: Routledge, Taylor & Francis Group.

Beck, J. (1995). *Cognitive therapy: Basics and beyond.* New York: Guilford Press.

Burns, D.D. (1999). *Feeling good: The new mood therapy* (Rev. ed.). New York: Harper Collins.

Leahy, R.L. (2003). *Cognitive therapy techniques: A practitioner's guide.* New York: Guilford Press.

Ledley, D.R., Marx, B.P., & Heimberg, R.G. (2005). *Making cognitive-behavioral therapy work: Clinical process for new practitioners.* New York: Guilford Press.

Sanders, D., & Wills, F. (2005). *Cognitive therapy: An introduction* (2nd ed.). London: Sage Publications.

# Hypnotherapy

Hypnotherapy is introduced to provide leverage to the psychological treatment of depression (Alladin, 2006) and to prevent relapses (Alladin, 2006a; Alladin & Alibhai, 2007). Hypnotherapy is specifically used to (a) induce relaxation, because 50% to 76% of depressed patients have comorbid anxiety (see Dozois & Westra, 2004); (b) reduce distraction; (c) maximize concentration; (d) facilitate divergent thinking; (e) amplify and expand experiences; (f) acquire sense of control; and (g) provide access to nonconscious psychological processes.

Cognitive hypnotherapy (CH) devotes four to six sessions to hypnotherapy. The first two or three sessions are devoted to (a) inducing relaxation, (b) producing somatosensory changes, (c) demonstrating the power of the mind, (d) expanding awareness, (e) strengthening the ego, (f) teaching self-hypnosis, and (g) offering posthypnotic suggestions. The remaining two to three hypnotherapy sessions focus on cognitive restructuring under hypnosis and unconscious exploration; these are described in Chapter 10. This chapter explores the seven hypnotherapeutic procedures that are the focus of the first two to three sessions.

## Relaxation Training

Various hypnotic induction techniques can be utilized to induce relaxation. I use the *relaxation with counting method* (see Gibbons, 1979) for inducing and deepening the hypnotic trance. I have chosen this technique because it is easily adapted for self-hypnosis training. One of the important goals of using hypnosis is to induce relaxation. Most depressed patients experience high levels of anxiety either due to comorbid anxiety (Dozois & Westra, 2004) or due to their negative view of the future and their low level of confidence in their abilities to handle life challenges. For these reasons, depressed patients benefit greatly from learning relaxation techniques. As discussed in Chapter 5, the majority of patients treated with CH in our studies (Alladin & Alibhai, 2007; Alladin, 2006, 2006a) indicated that the relaxation experience was empowering. It boosted their confidence to interrupt anxious sequences in their lives. Some of these patients went on to say that for the first time in their life, they were able to relax completely and replace their depressive feeling with good feeling. This is not surprising to hypnotherapists, who routinely observe such changes in their patients. For example, Yapko (2003) states: "I have worked with many people who actually cried tears of joy or relief in a session for having had an opportunity to experience themselves as relaxed, comfortable, and positive when their usual experience of themselves was one of pain and despair" (p. 106). The hypnotherapeutic script in Appendix 9A provides some examples of the types of hypnotic suggestions that can be utilized to induce a feeling of deep relaxation.

p 73

**Producing Somatosensory Changes**

Hypnosis is a powerful therapeutic tool for producing a variety of cognitive, somatic, perceptual, physiological, visceral, and kinesthetic changes under controlled conditions (Alladin, 2006). This process was described as *syncretic cognition* in Chapter 4. The hypnotic production and modulation of these changes provide depressed patients with dramatic proof that they can change their feeling and experience, thus providing hope that they can alter their depressive affect. In turn, this guides them to reconstruct their negative belief systems, creates a greater sense of self-efficacy and empowerment, redefines their long-held belief that depression is a permanent state, and establishes new confidence in their therapy. DePiano and Salzberg (1981) believe such positive experience in patients is partly related to the rapid and profound behavioral, emotional, cognitive, and physiological changes brought on by the induction of the hypnotic experience.

**Demonstrating the Power of the Mind**

Eye and body catalepsies, associated with the challenge to open eyes and get up from the chair or couch, are induced to demonstrate the power of the mind over the body. These demonstrations reduce scepticism over hypnosis, instill confidence in depressed patients that they can produce significant emotional and behavioral changes, and foster positive expectancy. In one report, I (Alladin, 2006) describes the case of Bob, a 55-year-old electronics engineer with recurrent major depressive disorder who was successfully treated with CH. Bob was very skeptical of the psychological treatment of depression because he believed his illness was caused by a chemical imbalance. The demonstration of the power of mind over body via eye and body catalepsies, provoked by challenging him to open his eyes and get out of the reclining chair, reduced his scepticism about hypnosis. He became a model patient, and his therapy sessions turned into "fascinating sessions" (Alladin, 2006, p. 180).

**Expansion of Awareness**

Hypnosis provides a powerful vehicle for expanding awareness and amplifying experience. Brown and Fromm (in Hammond, 1990, pp. 322–324) describe a technique called *enhancing affective experience and its expression*, which can be utilized to expand and intensify positive feelings by (a) bringing underlying emotions into awareness, (b) creating awareness of various feelings, (c) intensifying positive affect, (d) enhancing "discovered" affect, (e) inducing positive moods, and (f) increasing motivation. Such a procedure not only disrupts the depressive cycle but also helps to develop antidepressive pathways. The procedure involves bringing underlying emotions into consciousness, amplifying the experience, and then expressing or communicating the experience. The object of this procedure is to help depressed patients create, amplify, and express a variety of negative and positive feelings and experiences. This technique attempts to further reinforce the view that the depressive affect is not invariant.

To bring an underlying emotion into awareness, the hypnotized patient is told, "When I count from one to five . . . by the time you hear me say FIVE . . . you will begin to feel whatever emotion is associated with your [symptom or problem]." Then the patient is helped to amplify the affect by stating, "When I count slowly from one to five . . . as I count, you will begin to feel [symptom or problem] more and more intensely, so that when I reach the count of FIVE, you will feel it in your body as strongly as you can bear it. . . . Now notice what you feel, and you will be able to describe it to me." The procedure can be expanded by including past and future projection.

### Ego-Strengthening

Ego-strengthening suggestions are offered to depressed patients to increase self-esteem and optimize the effects of hypnotherapy. The enhancement of feelings of self-esteem and self-efficacy can provide a powerful tool in working with depressed patients. Bandura (1977) has provided experimental evidence that *self-efficacy*, the expectation and confidence of being able to cope successfully with various situations, is one of the key elements in the effective treatment of phobic disorders. Individuals with a sense of high self-efficacy tend to perceive themselves as being in control. If depressed patients can be helped to view themselves as self-efficacious, they will perceive the future as being hopeful. The most popular method for increasing self-efficacy within the hypnotherapeutic context is to provide ego-strengthening suggestions. The concept of "ego-strengthening" was coined and popularized by Hartland (1971). The principle behind ego-strengthening, according to Hartland, is to "remove tension, anxiety, and apprehension, and to gradually restore the patient's confidence in himself and his ability to cope with his problems." Hartland's ego-strengthening suggestions consist of generalized supportive suggestions to increase the patient's confidence, coping abilities, positive self-image, and interpersonal skills. He points out that patients must feel confident and strong enough to let go of their symptoms. Hartland recommends using ego-strengthening as a routine procedure in psychotherapy, before the direct removal of symptoms or hypnoanalysis, as this is likely to:

. . . pay handsome dividends. Not only will the patient obtain more rapid relief from his symptoms, but he will display obvious improvements in other ways. You will notice him becoming more self-reliant, more confident, and more able to adjust to his environment, and thus less prone to relapse. (p. 197)

Torem (1990) regards ego-strengthening as analogous to a medical setting in which a patient is first strengthened by proper nutrition, general rest, and weight gain before being subjected to radical surgery. We (Alladin & Heap, 1991, p. 58) consider ego-strengthening to be "a way of exploiting the positive experience of hypnosis and the therapist–patient relationship in order to develop feelings of confidence and optimism and an improved self-image." Hammond (1990) has expanded on the ego-strengthening techniques for enhancing self-esteem and self-efficacy by including direct and indirect suggestions, unconscious exploration, unconscious commitment, imagery training, time distortion, hypnotic conditioning, and posthypnotic suggestions. With depressed patients, I find verbatim ego-strengthening suggestions (see Appendix 9A) derived from Hartland (1971) and Hammond (1990) particularly effective when given following induction and deepening. However, to ensure credibility and acceptance of the ego-strengthening suggestions, it is of paramount importance to first induce a positive feeling and a "pleasant state of mind." The ego-strengthening suggestions must be crafted in such a way that they sound credible and logical to the patient. For example, rather than stating *"every day you will feel better,"* it is advisable to suggest *"as a result of this treatment, and as a result of you listening to your tape every day, you will begin to feel better."* This set of suggestions not only sounds logical, but improvement becomes contingent on continuing with the therapy and listening to the self-hypnosis tape daily (Alladin, 2006, 2006a).

When ego-strengthening or positive suggestions are repeated internally, they become embedded in the unconscious mind and begin to exert an automatic influence on feelings, thoughts, and behavior (Hartland, 1971; Hammond, 1990; Heap & Aravind, 2002). Therefore, ego-strengthening is incorporated into hypnotherapy to enhance a patient's self-confidence and self-worth (Heap & Aravind, 2002). I find (Alladin, 1992) that depressed patients tend to engage in negative self-hypnosis (NSH), and Araoz (1981) considers NSH to be the common denominator in all psychogenic problems. More recently, Nolen-Hoeksema and her colleagues (see Nolen-Hoeksema, 2002 for review) have provided empirical evidence that individuals who ruminate a great deal in response to their sad or depressed moods have more negative and distorted perceptions of the past, present, and future. These ruminators or "moody brooders" then become increasingly negative and hopeless in their thinking, resulting in protracted depressive symptoms.

Within the CH formulation, ego-strengthening suggestions are offered to counter the NSH. We (Alladin & Heap, 1991, p. 58) consider ego-strengthening to be "a way of exploiting the positive experience of hypnosis and the therapist–patient relationship in order to develop feelings of confidence and optimism and an improved self-image" in depressed patients.

**Posthypnotic Suggestions**

Before terminating the hypnotic session, posthypnotic suggestions are given to counter problem behaviors, negative emotions, and dysfunctional cognitions (NSH) or negative self-affirmations. Depressed patients tend to ruminate on negative self-suggestions, particularly after a negative affective experience (e.g., "I will not be able to cope"). This can be regarded as a form of posthypnotic suggestion, which can become part of the depressive cycle. Yapko (2003) regards posthypnotic suggestions to be a very necessary part of the therapeutic process if the patient is to carry new possibilities into future experience. Hence many clinicians use posthypnotic suggestions to shape behavior. For example, Clarke and Jackson (1983) regard posthypnotic suggestion to be a form of higher-order conditioning, which functions as positive or negative reinforcement to increase or decrease the probability of desired or undesired behaviors, respectively. They have successfully utilized posthypnotic suggestions to enhance the effect of in vivo exposure among agoraphobics.

To break the depressive cycle, it is very important to counter NSH. Here's an example of a posthypnotic suggestion specifically worded to counter NSH: "As a result of this treatment, as a result of you listening to your tape everyday...everyday you will become less preoccupied with yourself...less preoccupied with your feelings...and less preoccupied with what you think other people think about you. As a result of this, everyday you will become more and more interested in what you are doing and what is going on around you."

### Self-Hypnosis Training

At the end of the first hypnotherapy session, the patient is provided with an audiotape of self-hypnosis (consisting of the full script from Appendix 9A) designed to (a) create a good frame of mind, (b) offer ego-strengthening suggestions, and (c) provide posthypnotic suggestions. The homework assignment provides continuity of treatment between sessions and offers patient the opportunity to learn self-hypnosis. The self-hypnosis component of CH is designed to create positive affect and counter NSH via ego-strengthening and posthypnotic suggestions. The ultimate goal of psychotherapy is to help the depressed patient establish self-reliance and independence. Alman (2001) believes patients can achieve self-reliance and personal power by learning self-hypnosis. Yapko (2003) contends that the teaching of self-hypnosis and problem-solving strategies to patients allows them to develop self-correcting mechanisms that give them control over their lives. All the patients from the CH group from our study (Alladin & Alibhai, 2007) indicated that they derived benefits from their self-hypnosis tape in the form of time-out, relaxation response, and getting into the habit of positive self-hypnosis. The study showed that patients from the CH group continued to progress at follow-up, and their improvement was significantly greater than that of the CBT group, especially with the anxiety scores.

These results provide evidence that the self-hypnosis tape was helpful in the management of depression after the termination of the treatment. This has led me (Alladin, 2006a) to utilize self-hypnosis as an important modality in the prevention of relapse in depression (see Chapter 16).

### SUMMARY

This chapter described seven hypnotherapeutic procedures for breaking the depressive cycle, producing antidepressive experience, promoting self-confidence, and establishing positive expectancy. The empirical and theoretical rationale for the effectiveness of these hypnotherapeutic procedures with depression is discussed (Alladin & Alibhai, 2007). Clinicians are encouraged to standardize these procedures and validate the relative effectiveness of these procedures in the management of depression.

**REFERENCES**

Alladin, A. (1992). Depression as a dissociative state. *Hypnos: Swedish Journal of Hypnosis in Psychotherapy and Psychosomatic Medicine*, 19, 243–253.

Alladin, A. (2006). Cognitive hypnotherapy for treating depression. In R. Chapman (Ed.), *The clinical use of hypnosis with cognitive behavior therapy: A practitioner's casebook* (pp. 139–187). New York: Springer Publishing Company.

Alladin, A. (2006a). Experiential cognitive hypnotherapy: Strategies for relapse prevention in depression. In M. Yapko (Ed.), *Hypnosis and treating depression: Advances in clinical practice* (pp. 281–313). New York: Routledge, Taylor & Francis Group.

Alladin, A., & Alibhai, A. (2007). Cognitive hypnotherapy therapy for depression: An empirical investigation. *International Journal of Clinical and Experimental Hypnosis*, in press.

Alladin, A., & Heap, M. (1991). Hypnosis and depression. In M. Heap & W. Dryden (Eds.), *Hypnotherapy: A handbook* (pp. 49–67). Milton Keynes: Open University Press.

Alman, B. (2001). Self-care: Approaches from self-hypnosis for utilizing your unconscious (inner) potentials. In B. Geary & J. Zeig (Eds.), *The Handbook of Ericksonian psychotherapy* (pp. 522–540). Phoenix, AZ: The Milton H. Erickson Foundation Press.

Araoz, D.L. (1981). Negative self-hypnosis. *Journal of Contemporary Psychotherapy*, 12, 45–52.

Bandura, A. (1977). Self-efficacy: Toward a unifying theory of behavioral change. *Psychological Review*, 84, 191–215.

Brown, D.P., & Fromm, E. (1990). Enhancing affective experience and its expression. In D.C. Hammond (Ed.), *Hypnotic suggestions and metaphors* (pp. 322–324). New York: W.W. Norton.

Clarke, J.C., & Jackson, J.A. (1983). *Hypnosis and behavior therapy: The treatment of anxiety and phobias.* New York: Springer.

DePiano, F.A., & Salzberg, H.C. (1981). Hypnosis as an aid to recall of meaningful information presented under three types of arousal. *International Journal of Clinical and Experimental Hypnosis*, 29, 283–400.

Dozois, D.J.A., & Westra, H.A. (2004). The nature of anxiety and depression: Implications for prevention. In D.J.A. Dozois & K.S. Dobson (Eds.), *The prevention of anxiety and depression: Theory, research, and practice* (pp. 43–71). Washington, DC: American Psychological Association.

Gibbons, D.E. (1979). *Applied hypnosis and hyperempiria.* New York, Plenum Press.

Hammond, D.C. (Ed.) (1990). *Hypnotic suggestions and metaphors* (pp. 322–324). New York: W.W. Norton & Company.

Hartland, J. (1971). *Medical and dental hypnosis and its clinical applications* (2nd ed.). London: Bailliere Tindall.

Heap, M., & Aravind, K.K. (2002). *Hartland's Medical and Dental Hypnosis* (4th ed.). London: Churchill Livingstone.

Nolen-Hoeksema, S. (2002). Gender differences in depression. In I.H. Gotlib & C.C. Hammen (Eds.), *Handbook of depression*. New York: The Guilford Press.

Torem, M.S. (1990). Ego-strengthening. In D.C. Hammond (Ed.), *Hypnotic suggestions and metaphors* (pp. 110–112). New York: W.W. Norton & Company.

Yapko, M.D. (2003). *Trancework: An introduction to the practice of clinical hypnosis* (3rd ed.). New York: Brunner-Routledge.

## APPENDIX 9A

### Hypnotic Induction and Ego-Strengthening: Counting with Relaxation Method Induction

Close your eyes and make yourself as comfortable as you can. Now I am going to count ONE to TEN ... As I count ... with every count you will become more and more relaxed ... so that when I reach the count of TEN ... at the count of TEN you will be resting in a deep trance.

*ONE:*  Just continue to breathe gently ... in and out ... and as you concentrate on my voice you begin to relax ... relaxing very deeply as you continue to listen to my voice.

*TWO:*  You begin to feel a heavy and relaxing feeling coming over you as you continue to listen to my voice. And as you continue to breathe in and out ... you will begin to feel your arms relaxing ... your legs relaxing ... and your entire body relaxing completely.

*THREE:*  You begin to feel that heavy and relaxing feeling beginning to increase ... more and more ... and you are beginning to relax ... more and more ... relaxing deeper and deeper all the time as you continue to listen to my voice.

*FOUR:*  You can feel that heavy and relaxing feeling increasing ... more and more as you continue to listen to my voice. And as I continue to count, with every count ... that heavy and relaxing feeling will continue to increase more and more ... until it causes you to drift into a deep and pleasant trance.

*FIVE:*  Just notice ... progressively you are becoming more and more relaxed ... more and more at ease ... more and more comfortable ... so that when I reach the count of TEN you will be resting in a deep trance.

*SIX:*  Just listen to my voice as I continue to count ... and by the time I get to the count of TEN ... you will be resting in a deep and pleasant trance.

*SEVEN:*  You are beginning to drift slowly into a deep ... deep trance.

*EIGHT:*  Just notice you are becoming more and more comfortable ... more and more at ease ... more and more deeply relaxed ... so that when I reach the count of TEN, you will be resting in a deep trance.

*NINE:*  And every time you breathe in and out ... you are drifting slowly into a deep and pleasant trance ... drifting slowly ... into a deep and pleasant trance.

*TEN:*  Drifting slowly into a deep trance as you continue to listen to my voice ... as you continue to breathe in and out ... drifting deeper ... and deeper ... down ... and down ... into a deep and pleasant trance.

## Deepening the Trance

You are in such a deep hypnotic trance now...that your mind and your body feel calm and peaceful. And now I am going to help you to feel even more relaxed. In order to do this, I am going to count ONE to FIVE. When I reach the count of FIVE...at the count of FIVE...you will be resting in a deep...deep...very deep trance.

*ONE:* Just let yourself go...just let yourself relax...

*TWO:* Not doing anything...not trying anything...just letting go...no efforts...effortless...

*THREE:* Becoming heavier and heavier...or lighter and lighter...sinking deeper and deeper into a deep trance...

*FOUR:* At the same time feeling detached...very, very detached...your whole body feeling completely detached...drifting into a deeper and deeper trance...

*FIVE:* Letting yourself drift into a deeper and deeper trance...drifting deeper and deeper all the time as you continue to listen to my voice.

## Creating a Pleasant State of Mind

You have now become so deeply relaxed...and you are in such a deep...deep trance...that your mind and your body feel completely relaxed...completely at ease. And you begin to feel a beautiful sensation of peace and relaxation...tranquility and calm...flowing through your mind and body...giving you such a pleasant feeling...such a beautiful sensation...that you feel completely relaxed...completely at ease. Your mind and your body feel completely relaxed...and perfectly at ease...feeling peaceful...calm...comfortable...completely relaxed. Totally relaxed...drifting into a deeper and deeper trance as you continue to listen to my voice.

## Ego-Strengthening Suggestions

Just continue to enjoy these beautiful feelings...and as you continue to enjoy this feeling of deep relaxation.... I am going to repeat some helpful and positive suggestions to you...and since you are very relaxed and in such a deep hypnotic trance...your mind has become so sensitive...so receptive to what I say...so that every suggestion that I give you...will sink so deeply into the unconscious part of your mind...that they will begin to cause such a lasting impression there...that nothing will eradicate them. These suggestions from within your unconscious mind will help you resolve your difficulties. They will help you with your thinking...that is, they will help you to think more clearly, more objectively, more realistically, and more positively. They will help you with your feelings...that is, they will make you to feel less anxious, less upset, less depressed. They will also help you with your actions and your behaviors...that is, they will help you to do more and more things that are helpful to you, and you will do less and less things that are not helpful to you.

You are now so deeply relaxed, you are in such deep hypnotic trance...that everything that I say will happen to you...for your own good...will happen more and more. And every feeling that I tell you that you will experience . . . you will begin experience more and more. These same things will happen to you more and more often as you listen to your tape. And the same things will begin to happen to you just as strongly . . . just as powerfully . . . when you are at home . . . or at work or at school . . . or in any situation that you may find yourself in.

You are now so deeply relaxed . . . you are in such a deep hypnotic trance . . . that you are going to feel physically stronger and fitter in every way. At the end of the session . . . and every time you listen to your tape . . . you will feel more alert . . . more wide awake . . . more energetic. Every day as you learn to relax . . . you will become much less easily tired . . . much less easily fatigued . . . much less easily discouraged . . . much less easily upset . . . much less easily depressed.

Therefore, everyday as you learn to relax . . . your mind and your body will feel physically stronger and healthier . . . your nerves will become stronger and steadier . . . your mind will become calmer and clearer . . . you will feel more composed . . . more relaxed . . . and able to let go. You will begin to develop the tendency to ruminate less . . . to catastrophize less . . . therefore, you will become less worried . . . less anxious and less apprehensive . . . less easily upset . . . less easily depressed.

As you become more relaxed, less anxious, and less worried everyday . . . you will begin to take more and more interest in whatever you are doing . . . in whatever is going on around you . . . that your mind will become completely distracted away from yourself. You will no longer think nearly so much about yourself . . . you will no longer dwell nearly so much on yourself and your difficulties . . . and you will become much less conscious of yourself . . . much less preoccupied with yourself and your difficulties . . . much less preoccupied with your own feelings . . . and much less preoccupied with what you think others think of you.

As you become less preoccupied with yourself, less conscious of yourself . . . you will be able to think more clearly . . . you will be able to concentrate more easily. You will be able to give your whole undivided attention to whatever you are doing . . . to the complete exclusion of everything else. Even if some thoughts cross your mind, you will be able to concentrate on the task without being distracted. As a result of this, your memory will begin to improve . . . so that you begin to see things in their true perspective . . . without magnifying your difficulties . . . without ever allowing them to get out of proportion. In other words, from now on . . . whenever you have a problem, you will examine it objectively and realistically . . . and decide what you can and cannot do about it. If you cannot resolve the problem . . . you will accept it and come to terms with it. But if the problem can be resolved . . . then you will make a plan . . . or come up with some strategies to overcome it however long it may take. Therefore, from now on . . . whenever you have a problem you will become less emotionally upset and less overwhelmed by it. From now on you will begin to examine your difficulties like a scientist, that is, taking everything into consideration and then coming up with a plan. As a result of this new attitude . . . you will become emotionally less upset . . . less anxious . . . less agitated . . . and less depressed.

Every day...you will begin to feel all these things happening...more and more rapidly...more and more powerfully...more and more completely...so that...you will feel much happier...much more contented...much more optimistic in every way. And you will gradually become much more able to rely upon...to depend upon yourself...your own efforts...your own judgment...your own opinions. In fact...you will begin to feel much less need...to rely upon...or to depend...upon...other people.

**Termination**

Now...for the next few moments just let yourself relax completely...and continue to feel this beautiful sensation of peace...and relaxation...tranquility...and calm...flowing through your entire body...giving you such a pleasant...such a soothing sensation...that you feel so good...so at ease...that you feel a sense of well-being.

In a moment...when I count from ONE to SEVEN you will open your eyes...and will be alert...without feeling tired...without feeling drowsy. You will feel much better for this deep and pleasant hypnotic experience. You will feel completely relaxed both mentally and physically...and you will feel confident both in yourself and the future.

Now I am going to count ONE to SEVEN: ONE...TWO...THREE...FOUR...FIVE...SIX...SEVEN... Open your eyes...feeling relaxed, refreshed, and a sense of well being.

# Cognitive Hypnotherapy

Once the depressed patient becomes familiar with cognitive behavior therapy (CBT) and hypnotherapy, the next few sessions attempt to integrate cognitive and hypnotic strategies in the treatment. Specifically these sessions focus on (a) cognitive restructuring under hypnosis and (b) symbolic imagery techniques for dealing with a variety of emotional problems such as guilt, anger, fears, doubts, and anxieties. Before describing unconscious cognitive restructuring, the CBT methods of uncovering and restructuring core beliefs are first described.

## RESTRUCTURING CORE BELIEFS

As reviewed in Chapter 2, Beck (1976) proposed that each diagnostic condition is characterized by certain schemas or habitual patterns of thinking that represent vulnerability. Depressive schemas seem to reflect concerns about loss, failure, rejection, and depletion (Leahy, 2003). This approach to therapy focuses on assisting the patient to identify and modify his schema or core beliefs. Patients are coached to differentiate between surface or automatic cognitive distortions ("I can't do this") and deeper or enduring ("I'm a failure") negative cognitive structures (self-schemas). The therapist uses different strategies to restructure the deeper self-schemas. As discussed in Chapter 2, the term *schema* refers to enduring, deep cognitive structures or "templates" that are particularly important in structuring perceptions and building up "rule-giving" behaviors (Sanders & Wills, 2005). According to Sanders and Wills, schemas are:

- Unconditional
- Not immediately available to consciousness
- Latent, activated by triggering events
- Can be functional or dysfunctional, depending on the patient's life experience and cherished goals
- Compelling or noncompelling, depending on their influence on the patient's life
- Pervasive or narrow in the extent to which they influence the patient's life

A depressed person spirals down from surface thinking to dysfunctional assumption to core beliefs, all grounded in an early maladaptive schema (adapted from Sanders & Wills, 2005):

1. *Negative automatic thought:* "They don't care for me" (a high school teacher referring to her colleagues at a staff meeting). The thought states that the teachers at this specific meeting do not care for her. Despite the upset of this specific situation,

however, it is possible that other teachers in many other situations do care for her.

2. *Dysfunctional assumption:* "If I take my work seriously and try to be a good teacher, it may be possible for other teachers to care for me."

3. *Core belief:* "No one cares for me. No matter what I do, however hard I try to be a good teacher, no matter how much effort I put into pleasing my students and my colleagues, I don't seem to get anywhere, no one seems to care."

4. *Early maladaptive schema:* This patient's parents divorced when she was 9 years old. Although both parents had custody, she had to live with her grandparents because her father worked overseas and her mother was at school. She felt rejected, uncared for, and unloved by her parents. At school, she was teased and bullied for being overweight. She developed a profound sense of worthlessness, resulting in the deep belief that no one cares for her because she is unworthy.

Although interest is growing in the role of schemas as risk factors in depression, CBT usually adopts the principle of parsimony; that is, initially the work begins at the symptom level, particularly with automatic thoughts. Beck, et al. (1979) stress that "insight" work is not recommended during severe depression, because the patient is incapacitated by feeling of hopelessness and difficulty with concentration. Similarly, "working through" the depressive symptoms using cognitive techniques alone may also be counterproductive and may worsen negative feelings. Cognitive work becomes productive only after some of the most severe symptoms have lifted. Blackburn and Davidson (1995) estimate that approximately 75% of standard CBT for depression is directed at the symptom level, particularly working with behavioral responses to passivity and countering negative automatic thoughts. Only 25% of CBT is concerned with underlying issues and preventative work. Schema work or schema-focused therapy becomes a major focus of CBT when case conceptualization demands address underlying issues (e.g., in a complex case, or when the depression is comorbid with personality disorder) or when it is predicted that a depressed patient is at risk of relapse due to unaddressed underlying negative self-schemas.

The development of schema-focused therapy has undoubtedly expanded our understanding and treatment of depression. On the other hand, such a development raises some concerns, as echoed by Sanders and Wills (2005, p. 151):

We have observed that therapists from other disciplines are more likely to believe that core beliefs and early experience are where the action is. They tend to want to dive into these areas early on in therapy, neglecting to fully explore maintenance cycles and day-to-day aspects of the client's problems, perhaps feeling that they are not doing "real therapy" without bringing up the past.

Depressed patients can be extremely vulnerable when exposing and examining their core beliefs. Although the *downward arrow method* (described later) is a very simple CBT technique for uncovering core beliefs, it can lead to strong emotional consequences as a patient unmasks a strongly held, although such a belief has been unconscious. Sanders and Wills (2005, p. 152) caution that: "Unpacking a seemingly straightforward negative thought can lead to uncovering difficult and sensitive meanings, and if this is done too early in therapy, before the person is able to cope with the consequences, then he or she may end up feeling much worse." James (2001) and James and Barton (2004) therefore recommend that therapists think through the possible emotional reactions and consequences of accessing core beliefs. They suggest that hypotheses about core beliefs are brought on gradually and sensitively into the course of therapy rather than suddenly or confrontationally. It should also be noted that beliefs can be mood dependent. A person may consider herself useless and worthless when depressed, but when not depressed such core beliefs vanish. James, Southam, and Blackburn (2004) believe it may be "counterproductive" and "aversive" to dig for core beliefs when a person is not depressed. Moreover, they believe therapists must have sufficient skill and expertise, therapy time, and supervision to do this kind of work. For this reason, the circular feedback model of depression (CFMD) described in Chapter 4 places "symbolic transformation" further up in the cycle, although it has the potential to trigger the depressive cycle on its own. This position emphasizes that digging into core beliefs should come later in the course of therapy. Moreover, CH case formulation, which adopts the "stepped care" model (Davidson, 2000), provides a useful approach in deciding when and where to start working at a deeper level. The stepped care approach advocates delivering services in the most parsimonious way. The simplest intervention is adopted initially. More intensive and expensive forms of therapy are only used where there is clear evidence for their effectiveness and where they are likely to serve the patient's best interests. Sanders and Wills (2005) recommend avoidance of core-belief work with mild depression and single-episode problems. They believe core-belief work is most appropriate in the following situations:

- When there is clear trauma emerging from early or previous experience
- With deeper themes emerging strongly from the patient's history
- When early attempts to reduce symptoms have not worked
- When the patient requests long-term therapy focusing on early experience

Difficult issues should be uncovered only after a patient has learned some coping skills for dealing with these problematic situations. A good therapeutic relationship is central to schema-focused work because the therapist may choose to play a role in "limited reparenting" (Young, Klosko, & Weishaar, 2003), in which the therapist tries to offer a therapeutic relationship that counteracts the schema. However, such therapeutic reparenting should be approached with caution.

## UNCOVERING CORE BELIEFS WITH CBT

Beck (1976) believes that, to a large extent, both surface and core beliefs are semiunconscious; hence, he refers to them as being "automatic." Beck and other cognitive therapists have developed a variety of techniques for accessing and restructuring core beliefs.

The downward arrow method for uncovering core beliefs and the *circle of life technique* for restructuring core beliefs are described here. A technique for discovering the origin of the schema is also described.

### Downward Arrow Method

The downward arrow method is the most common CBT technique for uncovering core beliefs. An excerpt from a session with John, who logged the surface cognition *"I hate going to school"* in column B of the Cognitive Restructuring Form, shows how to get to a core belief by repeatedly questioning and asking for clarification:

*Therapist:* John, what do you mean by "I hate going to school?"

*John:* I don't like to be around people.

*Therapist:* What do you mean?

*John:* Well, I feel uneasy.

*Therapist:* What it is that makes you feel uneasy?

*John:* Well, people will notice that I am no good.

*Therapist:* What do you mean?

*John:* Well, I'm not as good as others.

*Therapist:* What do you mean?

*John:* I'm a failure.

*Therapist:* What do you mean?

*John:* I will never succeed because I'm no good. So what's the point of going to school?

### Circle of Life Technique

Once the core belief (in this case: "I'm no good, I'm a failure") is uncovered, several CBT techniques can be used to restructure them. I find the circle of life technique very effective in dealing with such core beliefs as "I'm a Failure," "I'm no good," "I'm useless," or "I'm bad." The next part of the transcript illustrates how the circle of life technique was utilized to help John restructure his core beliefs of "I am no good" and "I'm a failure."

*Therapist:* Let's see how we can help you with these deep beliefs that you have that you are "no good" and you are "a failure." Would you believe it if I say to you that a person can't be good or bad? (The therapist writes down on the top of a blank sheet of paper: Good/Bad; Success/Failure.)

*John:* Of course not. Some people are good, some people are bad.

*Therapist:* Would you believe me if I say to you a person can't be a success or a failure?

*John:* No.

*Therapist:* Let me show you why it's inaccurate to believe a person is either good or bad, or a success or a failure. Let's imagine this circle represents life (the therapist draws a large circle on the blank sheet of paper just below where earlier he wrote: Good/Bad; Success/Failure); of course, this is an oversimplification. We say we exist because we participate in hundreds of activities daily (the therapist fills the inner circle with about 20 large dots). Let's imagine each dot represents one activity and, as you can imagine, we participate in hundreds of activities every day. We go to school, we walk, we talk, we work, and so on. Do you agree?

*John:* Yes. You are right, we do many things everyday.

*Therapist:* That's right. We do many things in a day. Do you know of anyone who does everything very well?

*John:* No.

*Therapist:* Do you know of anyone who does everything badly?

*John:* No. I see what you mean. Not everyone does everything well or badly.

*Therapist:* That's right! No one does everything badly or very well. It's more accurate to say we all do some things well, and we do some things badly.

*John:* You are right. I never thought about it this way.

*Therapist:* Let's suppose I do some things badly (the therapist crosses three dots inside the circle). Does this make me a bad person?

*John:* No. You are still good at doing other things.

*Therapist:* That's right. I am still good at other things, although I mess up some of the things I do. Because I am not good with these things (therapist pointing to the three crossed out dots), it does not mean all the other activities that I am good at (the therapist pointing to the uncrossed dots) are totally wiped out.

*John:* It's so amazing. I never thought about it this way. Because I am a bit nervous when talking to people, it doesn't mean I am no good at anything. I thought because I feel nervous, I can't be a good person, I thought I must be a failure.

*Therapist:* I'm happy that you can relate to this, and you realize that you were thinking the wrong way.

*John:* I feel so relieved knowing what I was doing wrong.

*Therapist:* I'm glad now you know what to do. Similarly, a person can't be a success or a failure. We are all successful with some things, and we fail with some things.

*John:* I was convinced I was a failure because I could not do things as well as my friends.

*Therapist:* Are any of your friends successful with everything?

*John:* No. They can't be.

*Therapist:* That's right: They can't be. Just like you and I, your friends are successful with certain things, and they are not very good with other things.

*John:* I agree with you.

**Origin of Schemas**

At this point, the therapist can probe to discover the origin of the core belief. Discovering the origin helps the patient understand that he was not "born bad" but developed or learned such a schema through negative experience.

*Therapist:* John, what's the link? Where does this belief that you are "no good" or "a failure" come from?

*John:* As I told you in the first session, my father was very strict and demanding. He was never satisfied with whatever I did. I remember in Grade 9, I got 90s in every subject, except for math, in which I got 85. My father was mad that I did not get 90. At school I was shy so I used to be very quiet and, because of this, I got bullied and left out. I felt the kids did not want me. I began to believe I am no good. I even thought I was abnormal.

*Therapist:* So because your father and your peers at school undermined you, you started to believe you are no good, you were abnormal.

*John:* I remember on several occasions in Grade 10, I did not want to go to school. In the night, I used to lie in my bed, not sleeping, thinking of the next day. I hated being called "Shorty." People used to pick on me because I was short; I am still 5 foot 7. I even believed my father hated me because I was short.

*Therapist:* So you believed you are no good, you are abnormal because you were short. And what do you think of your height now?

*John:* I know I'm a bit short, but my height does not bother me now. But I still believe I'm a failure. But what you told about the Circle of Life made me realize I'm not a failure.

*Therapist:* I am glad to hear that. But let's recap. Now we know where your core beliefs come from. If you were to refer to the list of Cognitive Distortions from David Burns' book, what kinds of thinking errors are your core beliefs?

*John:* All-or-Nothing Thinking and Labeling.

*Therapist:* Excellent. But from now on, if the core beliefs come into your head that you are a failure, you are no good, how are you going to deal these thoughts?

*John:* I will remind myself that these are distorted way of thinking, and I will reason with them as you explained with the Circle of Life thing.

*Therapist:* Excellent. Do you think your father hates you?

*John:* No. I have already come to the realization that he did not hate me, but he was hard on me, the military type. My father was in the army.

*Therapist:* It seems you have already been doing some work with your emotional difficulties. Excellent work, John!

## RESTRUCTURING UNCONSCIOUS COGNITIVE DISTORTIONS

Very often in the course of CBT a patient is unable to access cognitions preceding certain negative emotions. Because hypnosis provides access to unconscious cognitive distortions and negative self-schemas, unconscious maladaptive cognitions can be easily retrieved and restructured under hypnosis. This is achieved by directing the patient's attention to the psychological content of an experience or situation. The patient is guided to focus attention on a specific area of concern and to establish the link between cognition and affect. Once the negative cognitions are identified, the patient is instructed to restructure the maladaptive cognitions and then to attend to the resulting (desirable) syncretic responses. For example, if a patient reports: "I don't know why I felt depressed at the party last week," the patient is hypnotically regressed back to the party and encouraged to identify and restructure the faulty cognitions until the patient can think of the party without being upset. Hypnosis also provides a vehicle whereby cognitive distortions below the level of awareness can be explored and expanded. I use three hypnotic strategies for restructuring cognitive distortions under hypnosis: (a) regression to the event triggering the negative affect, (b) regression to the original traumatic event, and (c) editing and deleting the unconscious file.

**Regression to the Activating Event**

While in a deep hypnotic trance state, the patient is suggested to imagine a situation that normally causes upset. The patient is instructed to focus on the emotional, physiological, and behavioral responses, and be aware of the associated dysfunctional cognitions. Encouragement is given to identify or "freeze" (frame by frame, like a movie) the faulty cognitions in terms of thoughts, beliefs, images, fantasies, and daydreams. Once a particular set of faulty cognitions is frozen, the patient is coached to replace it with more appropriate thinking or imagination, and then to attend to the resulting (desirable) "syncretic" (matrix of affective, cognitive, somatic, and behavioral responses) response. This process is repeated until the set of faulty cognitions related to a specific situation is considered to be successfully restructured.

**Regression to the Trauma**

This strategy is used when, during therapy, it becomes important to identify the origin of a core belief. I described the case of Rita, a 39-year-old housewife with a 10-year history of recurrent major depressive disorder who responded well to CH but continued to have symptoms of sexual dysfunction, which often served as a trigger for her depression (Alladin, 2006). Whenever her husband showed an interest in her, including in nonsexual scenarios, she would freeze and withdraw. Rita was "convinced there was something wrong with her at an unconscious level that might be affecting her sexual desire and sexual activity" (Alladin, 2006, pp.176–177). Hypnotic regression helped to bridge the link between her affect and her cognition. From the hypnotic regression, Rita was able to remember an incident when she was molested by her uncle when she was 7 years old. She had so much love and respect for her uncle that she became confused after the incident and concluded that "men are bad; I will never let them come near me." Once these core dysfunctional cognitions were identified, the circle of life technique was used to help her come to the understanding that not all men are bad. She was also encouraged under hypnosis to give herself permission to break her self-promise that she would never let a man touch her, because this promise was made while she was a child and totally confused.

**Editing and Deleting the Unconscious File**

A contemporary method of cognitive restructuring under hypnosis uses the metaphor of editing or deleting old computer files. This method is particularly appealing to children and adolescents. At the start of the session, the therapist and patient decide on which "file" of memories and perceptions the patient will work. While the patient is in a fairly deep state of hypnotic trance, she is instructed to become aware of "good feelings" (after ego-strengthening and amplification of positive feelings) and then directed to focus on personal achievements and successes (adult ego state). Attempts are made to get the patient to focus on the adult ego faculties of cognition, synthesis, integration, reality testing, and clear judgment. Once this is achieved, the patient is ready to work on modifying old learning and experiences. The patient is then instructed to imagine opening an old computer file that requires editing or deletion; she must edit or delete it, paying particular attention to dysfunctional cognitions, maladaptive behaviors, and negative feelings. By metaphorically deleting and editing the file, the patient is able to mitigate cognitive distortions, magical thinking, self-blaming, and other self-defeating mental scripts (i.e., NSH).

Other hypnotic uncovering or restructuring procedures such as affect bridge, age regression, age progression, and dream induction can also be used to explore and restructure negative self-schemas.

## SYMBOLIC IMAGERY TECHNIQUES

Depression can often be maintained by conscious or unconscious feeling of guilt and self-blame (old garbage). Various hypnotherapeutic techniques can be used to reframe those of the patient's past experiences that cause guilt or self-regret. Hammond (1990) describes several symbolic imagery techniques for dealing with guilt and self-blame. Hammond (1990) suggests that the hypnotic state facilitates a suspension of "generalized reality orientation," thus allowing the imagination to powerfully influence thoughts and feelings. Four symbolic imagery techniques for dealing with guilt and self-blame are briefly described. These techniques are normally used with depressed patients in the late phase of treatment, after the patient is sufficiently versed in CBT and hypnotherapy. Any of these techniques are introduced when the patient is in a fairly deep trance state.

### The Door of Forgiveness

The *door of forgiveness* technique was devised by Helen Watkins (1990) to help patients find their own self-forgiveness. The patient is asked to imagine walking down a corridor, at the end of which is the Door of Forgiveness. While walking, the patient notices several doors on either side of the corridor that she must pass before reaching the Door of Forgiveness. Some of these doors may appear familiar or meaningful to the patient. The patient is encouraged to open each meaningful door in turn and describe to the therapist what she observes inside the room. Here the idea is for the patient to resolve any experience or relationship out of the past that cause guilt before reaching the Door of Forgiveness.

Very often when a patient enters through a door, an emotional abreaction may occur. The therapist does not provide any interpretation and does not act as forgiver. The therapist's role is to provide direction and support.

### Dumping the Rubbish

Stanton (1990) uses the image of laundry to help a patient wash away her unwanted rubbish, such as fears, doubt, anxieties, and guilt. The patient is asked to imagine going to the laundry, filling the sink with water, opening a trap door from the head, and dumping the rubbish into the water, which become blacker and blacker. Finally, the patient imagines pulling out the plug from the sink and letting the inky water drain down the sink.

### Room and Fire

Here the image of a fireplace is used for burning unwanted garbage (Stanton, 1990). The patient is asked to imagine going down in the elevator from the tenth floor of a hotel to the basement. In the basement, there is a very cozy room with a large stone fireplace and a fire burning. The patient is asked to imagine throwing into the fire "Things you may not wish to keep in your life, such as fears, doubts, anxieties, hostilities, resentments, and guilts... one at a time, feeling a sense of release as they are transformed into ashes" (Stanton, 1990, p. 313).

### Red Balloon Technique

Hammond (1990) uses the hot air balloon as a metaphor for getting rid of unwanted negative emotions such as guilt and anger. The patient is asked to imagine walking up the hill with a large backpack. As the patient imagines climbing up the hill, the backpack gets heavier and heavier. Finally, the patient imagines coming across a moored hot air balloon with a gondola underneath, containing a large basket. The patient imagines throwing the burdensome, heavy, large backpack on the ground next to the gondola. Then the patient opens the backpack and tosses all the excessive and unwanted objects from it into the large basket in the gondola. Finally, the patient releases the balloon and, as the balloon flies away, the patient feels relieved for having unloaded all the unwanted garbage.

### SUMMARY

This chapter described both conscious and unconscious methods for accessing and restructuring core beliefs. Some techniques for uncovering the origin of schema were also described. The chapter recommends exercising parsimony and caution when working with core beliefs with depressed patients.

### REFERENCES

Alladin, A. (2006). Cognitive hypnotherapy for treating depression. In R. Chapman (Ed.), *The clinical use of hypnosis with cognitive behavior therapy: A practitioner's casebook* (pp. 139–187). New York: Springer Publishing Company.

Beck, A.T. (1976). *Cognitive therapy and emotional disorders*. New York: International University Press.

Beck, A.T., Rush, A.J., Shaw, B.F., & Emery, G. (1979). *Cognitive ther-apy of depression*. New York: Guilford Press.

Blackburn, I.M., & Davidson, K. (1995). *Cognitive therapy for depres-sion and anxiety* (2nd ed.). Oxford: Blackwell Scientific Publica-tions.

Davidson, G.C. (2000). Stepped care: Doing more with less? *Journal of Consulting and Clinical Psychology*, 68, 580–585.

Hammond, D.C. (Ed.) (1990). *Hypnotic suggestions and metaphors* (pp. 322–324). New York: W.W. Norton.

James, I.A. (2001). Schema therapy: The next generation, but should it carry a health warning? *Behavioral and Cognitive Psychother-apy*, 29, 401–407.

James, I.A., & Barton, S. (2004). Changing core beliefs with the con-tinuum technique. *Behavioral and Cognitive Psychology*, 32, 431–442.

James, I.A., Southam, L., & Blackburn, I.M. (2004). Schema revisited. *Clinical Psychology and Psychotherapy*, 11(4), 369–377.

Leahy, R.L. (2003). *Cognitive therapy techniques: A practitioner's guide*. New York: Guilford Press.

Sanders, D., & Wills, F. (2005). Cognitive therapy: An introduction (2nd ed.). London: Sage Publications.

Stanton, H.E. (1990). Dumping the "Rubbish." In Corydon D. Ham-mond (Ed.), *Handbook of hypnotic suggestions and metaphors* (p. 313). New York: W.W. Norton.

Watkins, H. (1990). The door of forgiveness. In Corydon D. Hammond (Ed.), *Handbook of hypnotic suggestions and metaphors* (pp. 313–315). New York: W.W. Norton.

Young, J., Klosko, J., & Weishaar, M.E. (2003). *Schema therapy: A practitioner's guide*. New York: Guilford Press.

# 11

# Developing Antidepressive Pathways

Chapter 9 described several hypnotherapeutic techniques for breaking the depressive cycle.

This chapter goes beyond disrupting and altering the depressive experience. The focus of this chapter is on describing the *positive mood induction* procedure for kindling the brain to enhance the development of antidepressive pathways. The development of such pathways will not only fortify the brain to withstand depressive symptoms, but will also prevent relapse and recurrence of future depressive episodes.

## POSITIVE MOOD INDUCTION

Although the hypnotic induction of relaxation, amplification of positive experience, expansion of awareness, and somatosensory changes described in Chapter 9 can kindle the brain, these procedures are not specifically utilized to develop antidepressive pathways. Their goals are to disrupt the depressive cycle and to alter the depressive affect. Positive mood induction is systematically devised to counter depressive pathways and to develop antidepressive pathways. Before describing the approach, the scientific underpinnings and theoretical rationale for developing antidepressive pathways are briefly reviewed.

I became interested in the antidepressive phenomena after reading the paper by Gary Schwartz and colleagues in the mid 1980s. Schwartz, Fair, Salt, Mandel, and Klerman (1976) provided electromyographic evidence to demonstrate that depressive pathways can be developed through conscious negative focusing. This finding led Schwartz (1984) to hypothesize that if it is possible to produce depressive pathways through negative cognitive focusing, then it should be possible to develop antidepressive or "happy pathways" by focusing on positive imagery. Although Schwartz's method of studying the relationship between cognition and brain functioning was primitive by current standards, his study was a landmark in the history of neuroscience. He was able to empirically demonstrate that cognition can mediate and alter brain responses. More recently, there has been a proliferation of electrophysiological and functional neuroimaging studies supporting the hypothesis that cognitive processes such guided imagery, cognitive restructuring, and hypnotic suggestions can alter brain functioning.

From their reviews of the imagery and sensory perception literature, Finke (1985) and Kosslyn (1988, 1994) have supplied strong evidence that the formation of a mental image in the brain resembles that of the actual perception of the corresponding external stimuli. Thus by the generation, manipulation, and scanning of mental images one can change the neural sensory processing mechanisms (for review, see Baer, Hoffman, & Sheikh, 2003). In the realm of CBT in the treatment of depression, Goldapple, Segal, Garson, Lau, Bieling, Kennedy, and Mayberg (2004) have provided functional neuroimaging evidence that cognitive restructuring produces specific cortical regional changes in treatment responders. Szechtman, Woody, Bowers, and Nahmias (1998) have demonstrated that when highly hypnotizable subjects claim to be experiencing hallucinations, the observed brain activity is extremely like that resulting from true sensory stimulation. Similarly, Kosslyn, Thompson, Constantini-Ferrando, Alpert, and Spiegel (2000) showed that hypnosis can modulate color perception. These investigators observed that hypnotized subjects were able to produce changes in brain function (measured by positron emission tomography [PET] scanning) similar to those that occur during visual perception. Rainville, Duncan, Price, Carrier, and Bushnell (1997) found the hypnotic suggestion of decreased pain to produce reduced regional cerebral blood flow in the anterior cingulate. In a separate controlled study, Rainville (see Bloom, 2005) demonstrated that words and images affect changes in regional blood flow in the brain structures associated with pain perception. Hypnotic suggestions also seem to suppress the *Stroop Conflict* (Raz, 2004; for review see Bloom, 2005). These findings support the claim that hypnotic suggestions can produce distinct neural changes correlated with real perception. From the foregoing evidence, it would not be unreasonable to infer that positive affect and images repeatedly induced by hypnosis and substantiated by regular personal training and exercise can produce some cortical changes in depressed patients.

Moreover, empirical evidence suggests that moods, both naturally occurring and experimentally manipulated, influence behavior (Gendolla, 2000; Baumeister & Vohs, 2004). Positive affect is the hallmark of well-being. Lyubomirsky, King, and Diener (2005) have provided extensive experimental, longitudinal, and correlational evidence to show that positive affect leads to adaptive approach and prosocial behaviors. Positive emotions also facilitate creative problem solving (Isen, 1999). People experiencing positive emotions are more open to processing new types of information and have greater flexibility (Fredrickson, 1998). Research also shows that positive emotions help to broaden the scope of attention (Fredrickson & Branigan, 2004). Furthermore, mood determines self-regulated behavior. Carver and Scheier (1990) have suggested that positive and negative moods serve as feedback about the person's progress in valued areas of life. Positive mood indicates that one is making satisfactory progress toward one's goals. Positive mood in depression may serve as a sign that one is making good progress in therapy towards recovery. Moreover, research shows that often people use current mood as a source of information for making evaluative judgments. People with positive mood tend to have a more favorable evaluation of their goal, while bad mood leads to less favorable evaluations (Schwarz & Strack, 1999). Additionally, King, Hicks, Krull, and Del Gaiso (2006) have provided empirical evidence that positive moods predispose individuals to feel life is meaningful and increase their sensitivity to the meaning or relevance of a situation.

In conclusion, it would appear that extensive empirical evidence suggests that positive affect (a) increases approach behavior, (b) provides greater flexibility in information processing, (c) broadens scope of attention, (d) directs goal behavior, (e) enhances favorable judgment, and (f) makes life appear more meaningful. In fact, all these are antidepressive behaviors. Repeatedly producing these antidepressive behaviors, concomitant with their positive affect, is bound to reduce depression.

The concept of *antidepressive pathways* is a metaphor; it denotes producing antidepressive experiences and their concomitant brain changes induced by hypnosis or by focusing on pleasant imageries. *Negative kindling* is the process of repeatedly eliciting negative affect and its concomitant neurochemical changes in the brain, whereas p*ositive kindling* is the process of producing antidepressive or positive experiences and its brain correlates. As discussed in Chapter 4, the kindling hypothesis has provided evidence for the development of increasing sensitization of the neurons in response to adverse life events in individuals who are prone to depression. Post (1992) has suggested that negative kindling may underlie the tendency for some depressed patients to suffer increasingly severe or refractory episodes of depression, or with passing time to require fewer provoking life events to relapse.

Segal, Williams, and Teasdale (1996) have integrated the kindling hypothesis with the cognitive theory of depression to explain the interplay between neuronal activity and cognitive processing in the development of risk and recurrence of depression. They posited that an elaborate network of depression-related material becomes activated when a person is depressed. This activation promotes the negative processing of stimuli, thus setting in motion a vicious cycle in which it becomes harder to activate cognitions to counteract negative thoughts. Within this framework, Segal, et al. (1996) conceptualize recurrence of depression to result from a lowered activational threshold for depressogenic structures or schemas in the presence of negative affect. Those with early negative life experiences also tend to experience a concomitant activation of negative thoughts. Activation of negative cognition increases accessibility to sad-related thoughts such as worthlessness and hopelessness, so that depressed patients begin to associate sadness with adversity. Gradually, depressogenic schemas become strongly associated and more generalized so that, over time, many more contexts can activate the depressed affect and depressive thinking. More recently, Monroe and Harkness (2005) refined the kindling hypothesis, providing an integrative model to explain the role of kindling in the recurrence of depression in the context of life stress.

Strong support for the kindling hypothesis was provided by Kendler, Thornton, and Gardner (2000) in a longitudinal study of over 2,000 community-based female twin pairs over 9 years, measuring depression and life-event severity during this period. They found a clear tendency for each episode of depression to be followed by an increased subsequent risk of a further episode of depression to be less strongly related to preceding life stress. Post

(1992) suggested that the increased vulnerability for recurrence of depression occurs at the neuronal level, and each episode leaves a neurobiological trace.

Thus, extensive empirical evidence suggests that directed cognition can produce neuronal changes in the brain and that positive affect can enhance adaptive behavior and cognitive flexibility. Within this theoretical and empirical context, the induction of positive mood in depression is considered to be a potent antidote for the depressive affect. Therefore, I regard the development of antidepressive pathways to be an important treatment component for depression. The next section describes training in positive mood induction.

## POSITIVE MOOD INDUCTION TRAINING

The positive mood induction technique for developing antidepressive pathways has five steps:

- Education
- Listing positive experiences
- Positive mood induction
- Posthypnotic suggestions
- Home practice

### Education

The patient is provided with a scientific rationale for producing antidepressive pathways. The findings from electromyographic and neuroimaging studies are described in lay terms. The kindling hypothesis is also discussed, and it is emphasized that *negative kindling* can produce depressive affect whereas *positive kindling* not only counteracts depressive pathways but also fortifies the brain by developing antidepressive pathways. Patients find the education component of the therapy very helpful.

### Listing Positive Experiences

The patient is helped to make a list of 10 to 15 pleasant or positive experiences. Because of their depression, some patients have difficulty making a list on their own. Therefore it is advisable to collaboratively work with the patient to compile the list rather than simply instructing the patient to make the list outside the treatment session.

### Positive Mood Induction

When in deep trance, the patient is instructed to focus on a positive experience from the list of positive experiences, which is then amplified with assistance from the therapist. The technique is very similar to enhancing affective experience and its expression, described under "Expansion of Awareness" in Chapter 9. However, to develop antidepressive pathways, more emphasis is placed on producing somatosensory changes in order to induce more pervasive concomitant physiological changes. The procedure is repeated with at least three positive experiences from the list of pleasant experiences. The script below provides some examples of the kinds of hypnotic suggestions that can be used for developing antidepressive pathways. Sarah is an 18-year-old high school student who had a major depressive episode when she was 16 years old. After a short hospital admission, Sarah was treated as an outpatient. She made good recovery using combined antidepressant medication and CBT. However, Sarah continued to have some residual symptoms, such as a sense of sadness, lack of pleasure, and feeling lethargic, although she continued to be on a prophylactic dose of selective serotonin reuptake inhibitor (SSRI). Because of these feelings, Sarah was not motivated to do most things young adults would do. Sarah held the belief that she would not enjoy doing anything if she did not feel motivated to do it. She equated motivation with pleasure. The positive mood induction technique was used to create positive feelings and to help her develop antidepressive pathways. Sarah did not have much difficulty making up a list of 14 pleasant experiences; one of them included having a barbecue with her friend Nikki and her family, in their back garden, in Acapulco, Mexico.

When working with the positive mood induction procedure, it is important to keep close rapport with the patient. The therapist should not assume he understands what the patient is experiencing; it is advisable for the therapist to set up ideomotor signaling before starting the procedure.

*Therapist:* You are doing very well (*while she was in a deep trance*). Just continue to enjoy this beautiful sensation of peace and tranquility, relaxation and calm flowing through your mind and body...giving you such a pleasant feeling...such a soothing sensation...that you feel you are drifting into a deeper and deeper hypnotic trance. And now I would like you to go back in time and place in your mind to when you were having a barbecue at Nikki's back garden in Acapulco (*pause*). Can you imagine yourself being there?

(*Sarah nods yes.*)

*Therapist:* Now, I would like you to become aware of the place where the barbecue was held. You may remember the garden (*visual accessing*), the size of the garden, the landscaping of the garden, the plants, the trees, the flowers. Remember all the details about the garden that you can. Can you imagine the full description of the garden?

(*Sarah nods yes.*)

Very good! Now can you remember the details of the barbecue pit?

(*Sarah nods.*)

Now you may remember all the people who were there...their names...the way they were dressed...and other details about the people...especially you may remember how you were dressed...and how Nikki was dressed up.

(*Sarah nods.*)

As you remember the details, you feel you are getting more and more absorbed, becoming more and more relaxed...drifting into a deeper and deeper trance (*the imagery is used to deepen the trance and to increase relaxation*).

Now you may remember the weather (*induction of kinesthetic feeling*)...whether it was hot, mild, or breezy. Was it a hot day?

*(Sarah nods; the therapist made this assumption because Sarah tactile told the therapist that she visited Acapulco during the summer.)*

You may remember the sun shining, you may remember how hot it was... maybe beginning to remember how warm you felt... how hot you felt... you may feel the warm sensation.

*(Sarah nods.)*

And as you remember the feeling of warmth, just notice you are becoming more and more relaxed, more and more warm... drifting into a deeper and deeper trance, and soon you may feel you are there, as if you are re-experiencing everything.

Now perhaps you may remember the smell (*olfactory accessing*) of the garden, the smell of the food. First, let's focus on the garden. You may remember the smell of the flowers, maybe the lawn was freshly mowed... you may remember the smell of the freshly cut lawn. You may remember the aroma of the food being barbecued.

*(Sarah nods.)*

You may begin to feel your mouth watering (*gustatory accessing*).

*(Sarah nods.)*

And you may remember the freshly barbecued food you ate... remembering the flavor of the good food you had. And the cool and tasty drinks you had. How good it felt eating the fresh food and drinking the very tasty drinks. As you remember these details, just notice you are becoming more and more absorbed... feeling as if you are there. As if you are re-experiencing everything... drifting into a deeper and deeper trance... savoring the fresh food, the tasty drinks.

*(Sarah continues to nod agreement to these sensory accessing clues.)*

Maybe now you remember all the good feelings you had (*accessing affect; affect is accessed last because it is easier to remember and feel affect when all the senses are already involved in the situation*)... the good feelings you experienced.

*(Sarah nods.)*

Remember how good it felt being with your friend and enjoying the barbecue, enjoying the company. Just become aware of all the good feelings you are feeling (*bringing the dissociated experience to the present in order to amplify the sensory and affective experiences*)... feeling very, very relaxed (*the voice is modulated to get a response from Sarah and she nods.*) Feeling calm, peaceful (*pause; Sarah nods*)... happy and pleased. Just stay with these feelings for the next few moments... enjoying the good feelings... feeling good... feeling happy. Do you feel all these? (*Sarah nods.*)

**Posthypnotic Suggestions**

Before terminating the trance, the patient is given posthypnotic suggestions about "positive focusing" and "whenever possible, imagine playing one of the pleasant experiences in your mind." The following posthypnotic suggestions were given specifically about the barbecue:

*Therapist:* Every time you think of Nikki's barbecue, you will experience these same feelings, just as strongly, just as fully, just as completely as if you are there... and with practice it will become easier and easier for you to become absorbed in the situation.

### Home Practice

Home practice is an essential part of the training. It is emphasized to the patient that home practice will make it easier to access the pleasant experiences associated with their list, and it will induce positive affect that will strengthen the antidepressive pathways and weaken the depressive pathways. The patient is advised to practice using their list at least twice a day, and instructed to focus on each pleasant experience for about 1 minute.

## SUMMARY

This chapter briefly reviewed the relationship between cognition and brain responses and the influence of positive mood on behavior. Within this empirical context, the positive mood induction technique was devised to develop antidepressive pathways. The positive mood induction technique provides a self- and therapist-guided procedure for kindling the brain positively. Since negative kindling can produce depressive pathways, then it is not unreasonable to hypothesize that repetitive positive kindling will develop antidepressive pathways. Indirect evidence from neuroimaging studies with CBT suggests that cognitive manipulation can produce cortical changes.

## REFERENCES

Baer, S.M., Hoffman, A.C., & Sheikh, A.A. (2003). Healing images: Connecting with inner wisdom. In A.A. Sheikh (Ed.), *Healing images: The role of imagination in health* (pp. 141–176). New York: Baywood.

Baumeister, R.F., & Vohs, K.D. (Eds.) (2004). *Handbook of self-regulation: Research, theory, and applications.* New York: Guilford.

Bloom, P.B. (2005). Advances in neuroscience relevant to clinical hypnosis: A clinician's perspective. *Hypnos, 32,* 17–23.

Carver, C.S., & Scheier, M.F. (1990). Origins and functions of positive and negative affect: A control-process view. *Psychological Review, 97,* 19–35.

Finke, R.A. (1985). Theories relating mental imagery to perception. *Psychological Bulletin, 98,* 236–259.

Fredrickson, B.L. (1998). What good are positive emotions? *Review of General Psychology, 2,* 300–319.

Fredrickson, B.L., & Branigan, C. (2004). Positive emotions broaden the scope of attention and thought-action repertoires. *Cognition & Emotion, 19,* 313–332.

Gendolla, G.H.E. (2000). On the impact of mood on behavior: An integrative theory and review. *Review of General Psychology, 4,* 378–408.

Goldapple, K., Segal, Z., Garson, C., Lau, M., Bieling, P, Kennedy, S., & Mayberg, H. (2004). Modulation of cortical-limbic pathways in major depression: Treatment-specific effects of cognitive behavior therapy. *Archives of General Psychiatry, 61,* 34–41.

Isen, A.M. (1999). On the relation between affect and creative problem solving. In S.R. Russ (Ed.), *Affect, creative experience, and psychological adjustment* (pp. 3–17). Philadelphia: Taylor & Francis.

Kendler, K.S., Thornton, L.M., & Gardner, C.O. (2000). Genetic risk, number of previous depressive episodes, and stressful life events in predicting onset of major depression. *American Journal of Psychiatry*, 158, 582–586.

King, L.A., Hicks, J.A., Krull, J.L., & Del Gaiso, A.K. (2006). Positive affect and the experience of meaning of life. *Journal of Personality and Social Psychology*, 90, 179–196.

Kosslyn, S.M. (1988). Aspects of cognitive neuroscience of mental imagery. *Science*, 240, 1621–1626.

Kosslyn, S.M. (1994). *Image and brain*. Cambridge, MA: MIT Press.

Kosslyn, S.M., Thompson, W.L., Costantini-Ferrando, M.F., Alpert, N.M., & Spiegel, D. (2000). Hypnotic visual illusion alters color processing in the brain. *American Journal of Psychiatry*, 157, 1279–1284.

Lyubomirsky, S., King, L., & Diener, E. (2005). The benefits of frequent positive affect: Does happiness lead to success? *Psychological Bulletin*, 131, 803–855.

Monroe, S.M., & Harkness, K.L. (2005). Life stress, the "kindling" hypothesis, and the recurrence of depression: Considerations from life stress perspectives. *Psychological Review*, 112, 417–445.

Post, M.I. (1992). Transduction of psychosocial stress into the neurobiology of recurrent affective disorder. *American Journal of Psychiatry*, 149, 999–1010.

Rainville, P., Duncan, G., Price, D., Carrier, B., & Bushned, M. (1997). Pain affect encoded in human anterior cingulate but somatosensory cortex. *Science*, 277, 968–971

Raz, A. (2004). Atypical attention: Hypnosis and conflict reduction. In M.I. Posner (Ed.), *Cognitive neuroscience of attention* (pp. 420–429). New York: Guilford Publications.

Schwarz, N., & Strack, F. (1999). Reports of subjective well-being: Judgmental processes and their methodological implications. In D. Kahneman, E. Diener, & N. Schwarz (Eds.), *Well-being: The foundations of hedonic psychology* (pp. 61–84). New York: Russell Sage Foundation.

Schwartz, G. (1984). Psychophysiology of imagery and healing: A systems perspective. In A.A. Sheik (Ed.), *Imagination and healing* (pp. 35–50). New York: Baywood.

Schwartz, G., Fair, P.L., Salt, P., Mandel, M.R., & Klerman, G.L. (1976). Facial muscle patterning in affective imagery in depressed and non-depressed subjects. *Science*, 192, 489–491.

Segal, Z.V., Williams, J.M., Teasdale, J., & Gemar, M. (1996). A cognitive science perspective on kindling and episode sensitization in recurrent affective disorder. *Psychological Medicine*, 26, 371–380.

Szechtman, H., Woody, E., Bowers, K.S., & Nahmias, C. (1998). Where the imaginal appears real: A positron emission tomography study of auditory hallucinations. *Proceedings of the National Academy of Sciences*, 95, 1956–1960.

# Breaking Ruminative Pattern

As discussed in Chapter 2, Abramson and his colleagues (Abramson, Alloy, Hankin, Haeffel, MacCoon, & Gibb, 2002) have examined the relationship between cognitive vulnerability and Beck's theory of depression. Within the context of their cognitive vulnerability-stress model of depression, they studied the role of rumination. They found cognitive vulnerability to underlie the tendency to ruminate negatively, and they posited that cognitively vulnerable individuals are at high risk of engaging in rumination. Depressive rumination involves the perpetual recycling of negative thoughts (Wenzlaff, 2004). There is evidence that negative rumination leads to (a) negative affect, (b) depressive symptoms, (c) negatively biased thinking, (d) poor problem-solving, (e) impaired motivation and inhibition of instrumental behavior, (f) impaired concentration and cognition, and (g) increased stress and problems (for review, see Lyubomirsky & Tkach, 2004). Depressive ruminators are caught in a vicious cycle. Due to their rumination they become keenly aware of the problems in their lives, but at the same time they are unable to generate good solutions to those problems. Therefore, they feel hopeless about being able to change their lives (Nolen-Hoeksema, 2004).

Various approaches for treating rumination are described in the literature. They include thought stopping, in vivo and imaginal exposure, systematic desensitization and relaxation training, CBT, metacognitive therapy, mindfulness meditation, distraction therapy, and attention training therapy (Purdon, 2004). With depressive rumination, distraction therapy, CBT, and attention training therapy have been effective to some extent. Purdon (2004, pp. 221–222), from her review of the effectiveness of distraction therapy with depression concludes: "Suppression of depression-related thoughts appears to be somewhat successful in the short term, but these efforts may be highly vulnerable to disruption and therefore rather inefficient as a long-term strategy for managing depressive rumination." The lack of enduring effectiveness of distraction therapy can be attributed to two main causes: (a) the research on thought suppression shows that distraction or suppression leads to a rebound of thought occurrences once control efforts have ceased (e.g., Wegner, Schneider, Carter, & White, 1987); and (b) because negative ruminations are influenced by negative core beliefs (cognitive vulnerability), if these core beliefs are not corrected, the surface ruminations are likely to remain refractory (e.g., Rachman, 1997). Instead of thought suppression, a more positive, constructive method is to distract from the thoughts mindfully; that is, the mind is gently moved on to alternative, positive thoughts or images, seeing any intrusive thoughts as clouds across the field of vision or other imagery. This procedure is akin to detached mindfulness (see Chapter 15).

The effectiveness of CBT with depressive rumination has been modest. Although CBT is well established as the most effective psychological treatment for overcoming depression, its focus is on the cognitive triad, not on depressive rumination, because ruminative styles of thinking have not been given prominence in either the CBT model of depression or in the treatment of depression. In therapy, the focus of CBT has largely been on modifying the *content* of negative automatic thinking related to the cognitive triad, rather than focusing on the *process of negative thinking*. This bias in therapy may partially account for the large proportion of depressed patients who do not respond to CBT or who relapse following treatment. In other words, traditional CBT challenges the content or output of thoughts. Many clinicians (e.g., Wells and Papageorgiou, 2004) believe CBT would be more effective if it were to address processes or metacognitive beliefs, that is, how people arrive at what they "know." The concept of metacognition includes an analysis of how an individual's thinking about his thinking plays a key role in the development of psychological problems. For example, the patient who is depressed about everything has numerous negative, depressive thoughts. What is of interest is not simply the content and meaning of specific thoughts, but the meaning of thinking in this particular way.

Papageorgiou and Wells (2001) distinguish depressive rumination from negative automatic thoughts. They regard rumination as a coping strategy that exacerbates depression in the same way that anxious rumination (worry) serves to maintain anxiety. They interviewed depressed individuals about their rumination and found depressed people to hold positive views of their rumination. Depressed patients believe that their ruminations are helpful for solving problems, gaining insight, identifying potential triggers and causes, preventing future mistakes, and prioritizing important tasks. Unfortunately, because these ruminations are negative and unconstructive, they play a major role in the development, persistence, and relapse of depression. These findings highlight the necessity for restructuring these underlying beliefs or metacognitions. Understanding and correction of these metacognitive beliefs about the ruminations will likely decrease the erroneous use of rumination for problem solving, which will lead to a reduction of depressive symptoms. The *reasoning and attention switching* procedure for treating depressive rumination described in this chapter is based on these theoretical rationales and empirical findings.

Few treatments or techniques have been directly targeted at treating rumination in depression. The most structured and systematic treatment for depressive rumination, *attention training therapy* (ATT), has been developed by Wells (Wells, 1990; Wells & Papageorgiou, 2004). Single case studies have shown that ATT is helpful for a number of problems including health anxiety and major depression (see Wells & Papageorgiou, 2004). Similarly, I (Alladin, 1994, 2006), as part of my cognitive hypnotherapy package, have developed *thought stopping and attention switching* for dealing with depressive rumination. Because the focus of this technique has been on distraction, in the light of the recent findings that thought suppression leads to an increase in rumination, the technique has been revised and labeled *reasoning and attention switching* (RAAS).

## REASONING AND ATTENTION SWITCHING

In worry and rumination, the focus of attention is almost exclusively on negative thinking, and depressed individuals report being "lost in thought" and "out of touch with what else is going on" (Sanders & Wills, 2005, p. 119). RAAS provides a training and treatment procedure for decreasing depressive rumination and enabling the depressed person to become more flexible in what he attends to. RAAS is derived and adapted from ATT, described by Wells and his colleague (Wells, 1990; Wells & Papageorgiou, 2004) and *thought stopping and attention switching* developed by Alladin (1994, 2006). There are five phases for learning RAAS:

- Education
- Exploration of the advantages and disadvantages of rumination
- Attention training
- Restructuring metacognitive beliefs
- Home practice

### Education

The aim of the education phase is to help the patient understand the rationale for controlling depressive ruminations. The patient is helped to understand the association between a negative style of thinking and the triggering of depression. The role of metacognition or ruminative thinking in the exacerbation and maintenance of depression is highlighted.

### Advantages and Disadvantages of Rumination

The patient is encouraged to talk about the advantages of the depressive rumination. This approach facilitates the eliciting of positive metacognitive beliefs attached to depressive rumination. I find the comparison with smoking helpful as a starting point:

*Therapist:* When you talk to people who have been smoking for a long time, you learn that they derive many benefits from smoking. It helps them relax, distracts their minds from worries, and gives them something to do when they are bored. What are your reasons for ruminating when you feel depressed?

Wells and Papageorgiou (2004) have identified the following positive beliefs about rumination from their depressed patients:

- Helps to find ways of dealing with problems
- Helps to cope with depression in the future
- Helps the patient discover what is wrong with him
- Prevents the patient forgetting important people or events
- Keeps the person is in touch with reality
- Guards them against the dangers of thinking too positively (i.e., guards them against disappointment)

If a patient does not mention any one of these reasons, the therapist can go down the list and ask: "Does this apply to you?"

Once the patient has the opportunity to process the "positive" metacognitive beliefs, the therapist explores the disadvantages of the ruminative beliefs:

*Therapist:* As we mentioned before, people derive some benefits from smoking, but unfortunately it has some disadvantages. Can you think of the disadvantages?

After the patient has listed the disadvantages of smoking, the therapist adds: "Now let's examine the downside of rumination when depressed."

The therapist assists the patient in identifying the disadvantages of rumination, and these disadvantages are reinforced and elaborated on until they outweigh the advantages. Wells and Papageorgiou (2004) list the following disadvantages of rumination:

- Biased and focuses on negatives
- Often does not lead to solutions
- Intensifies negative mood
- Encourages a negative view of the whole self
- Interferes with focusing on outward tasks
- Makes one appear withdrawn
- Has a negative impact on others
- Is unproductive and impairs concentration
- Interferes with sleep
- Increases negative outlook

## Attention Training

Because depressed patients have difficulty interrupting self-focused rumination, training in attention switching is required. (Wells, 1990; Wells & Papageorgiou, 2004) has developed ATT for this purpose. The attention training (AT) described here is adapted from Wells.

After discussing the rationale, advantages and disadvantages of depressive rumination, and any concerns the patient might raise about the credibility of the treatment, the therapist introduces AT. AT consists of six components:

Orientation
Selective attention
Rapid attention switching
Simultaneous attention
Hypnotic reinforcement
Home practice

### *Orientation*

AT can be introduced by stating: "Now that we have a good understanding of why it is important to control negative rumination, I am going to teach you a technique that will give you confidence in controlling your rumination. The technique involves learning to pay attention to different sounds and developing the ability to increase flexibility over attention."

### *Selective Attention*

Selective attention involves focusing on selected sounds. The script here, adapted from Wells (2000, pp. 145–146) and Wells and Papageorgiou (2004, pp. 266–267), illustrates how the procedure can be introduced to the depressed patient:

*Therapist:* I am going to ask you to focus on the sound of my voice. Pay close attention to the sound of my voice, no other sound matters. Try to give all your attention to the sound of my voice. Ignore all the other sounds around you. Other sounds are not important, focus only on the sounds of my voice, only on the sounds of my voice.

Now I would like you to focus on the tapping sound (*therapist taps on his desk*). Focus only on the tapping sound, no other sounds matter (*therapist continues to tap*). Closely monitor the tapping sound. If your attention begins to stray or is attracted by other sounds, refocus all your attention to the tapping sound (*therapists continues to tap*), to the tapping sound only. Monitor the sound closely; filter out all other sounds for they are not important. Continue to monitor the tapping sound, focusing all your attention on the tapping sound. Try not to be distracted, continue to focus on the tapping sound.

Now we are going to focus on the sound of the clock on the wall. Focus all your attention on the ticking of the clock. No other sounds matter. Just focus on the sound of the clock (*therapist pauses*). The other sounds don't matter, focus on that sound, paying close attention to the sound of the clock, not allowing yourself to be distracted (*therapist pauses*). This is the most important sound, nothing else matters, give all your attention to this sound. If your attention strays or you become attracted to other sounds, refocus all your attention to the sound of the clock. Focus on the sound of the clock only, giving all your attention to this sound, not allowing yourself to be distracted (*therapist pauses*).

### *Rapid Attention Switching*

Rapid attention switching requires shifting attention between different sounds. This part of the training provides confidence in the ability to switch attention rapidly from one source of attention to another.

*Therapist:* Now that you have been able to identify and focus on different sounds, I would like you to rapidly shift your attention between the different sounds as I call them out (*therapist pauses*). First, focus on the sounds of my voice, no other sound matters, giving your full attention to the sound of my voice.

Now switch on to the tapping sound (*therapist taps on his desk*), focusing on the tapping sound, no other sound matters, focusing all your attention to the tapping (*therapist continues to tap*).

Now switch to the sound of the clock, paying attention to the ticking of the clock, no other sound matters, giving all your attention to the sound of the clock (*therapist pauses*).

Now focus again on the sound of my voice. Focusing on my voice alone, not allowing your attention to be distracted.

### *Simultaneous Attention*

Simultaneous attention involves paying attention to different sounds simultaneously. Wells (1990) refers to this part of the training as "divided attention." This term is not used here to avoid confusion with Hilgard's (1974, 1977) concept of divided attention described in Chapter 3.

*Therapist:* Now we are going to expand your attention, so that your attention is broadened, so that you will be able to focus on many sounds at the same time. Become aware of all the sounds in the room (*therapist taps on his desk*), the tapping sound, the ticking of the clock, the sound of my voice, and any other sounds you may be aware of. Try to hear all the sounds at the same time, focusing on all the sounds. You may count the number of sounds you hear at the same time.

### Hypnotic Reinforcement

The AT procedure can be repeated following a formal hypnotic induction, or focusing on the sounds alone can be utilized to induce and deepen the hypnotic trance. For example: "As you listen to my voice, you feel you are becoming more and more relaxed" or "As you listen to the sound of tapping, notice you are drifting into a deeper and deeper trance." Repetition of the AT procedure under hypnosis makes the training more experiential, and the pairing of the sounds with relaxation reinforces a positive conditioned response to the sounds.

### Homework Practice

As homework, the patient is encouraged to devote 10 to 15 minutes, twice a day, to practicing AT. This is also reinforced as posthypnotic suggestion before terminating the trance. It is important for the therapist to monitor the progress and address any obstacles or difficulty that the patient may be encountering when practicing AT.

### Restructuring Metacognitive Beliefs

As indicated earlier, depressed patients have a set of metacognitive beliefs that reinforce their negative ruminations. It is important not to simply identify these metacognitions, but to also help the patient modify them. Based on his studies of obsessional rumination, Rachman (1997, 1998) argues that attention switching sustains the frequency of the obsessions and the erroneous beliefs about the meaning (metacognition) of the obsession. Guided by this research and the conclusion reached by Purdon (2004) that distraction therapy is not efficient as a long-term strategy for managing depressive rumination, cognitive restructuring of the depressive metacognitions is considered a very important component of RAAS. Since negative ruminations are influenced by negative core beliefs (cognitive vulnerability), if these core beliefs are not corrected, the surface ruminations are likely to remain refractory. The cognitive restructuring techniques described in Chapter 9 can be used to restructure the metacognitive beliefs. Papageorgiou and Wells (2001) have identified themes of mental breakdown, ineffectiveness, inferiority, and vulnerability to psychological disorder to be associated with depressive rumination. They believe these themes underlie the tendency for depressed patients to catastrophize minor symptoms of depression. Therapists should be alert to these themes, and they should be identified and addressed in therapy.

It is also helpful for the depressed patient to utilize the mindfulness approach described in Chapters 15 and 16. The procedure for *recognizing bias in thinking* described in Chapter 16 can also be useful in recognizing and countering distorted thinking (also see Alladin, 2006a, p. 306). For example, if a patient becomes aware of "disqualifying the positive," she can remind herself that "Positives too count—no excuses." Recognizing distorted thinking and counteracting it is akin to catching and halting negative self-hypnosis.

## SUMMARY

This chapter discussed the role of negative rumination as a risk factor in the development of depression and its importance in the triggering, exacerbation, and maintenance of depressive affect. RAAS, based on theoretical and empirical rationale, provides a systematic and structured approach for the management of depressive rumination. To enhance the effectiveness of this treatment approach, RAAS combines attention training with cognitive restructuring of the metacognitive beliefs that underlie the depressive rumination. There is some evidence that attention training is effective with depressive rumination. However, more research is required in this neglected, but important, area of depression.

## REFERENCES

Abramson, L.Y., Alloy, L.B., Hankin, B.L., Haeffel, G.J., MacCoon, D.G., & Gibb, B.E. (2002). Cognitive-vulnerability – Stress models of depression in a self-regulatory and psychobiological context. In I.H. Gotlib & C.L. Hammen (Eds.), *Handbook of depression* (pp. 268–294). New York: Guilford Press.

Alladin, A. (1994). Cognitive hypnotherapy with depression. *Journal of Cognitive Psychotherapy: An International Quarterly*, 8(4), 275–288.

Alladin, A. (2006). Cognitive hypnotherapy for treating depression. In R. Chapman (Ed.), *The clinical use of hypnosis in cognitive behavior therapy: A practitioner's casebook* (pp. 139–187). New York: Springer Publishing Company.

Alladin, A. (2006a). Experiential cognitive hypnotherapy: Strategies for relapse prevention in depression. In M. Yapko (Ed.), *Hypnosis and treating depression: Advances in clinical practice* (pp. 281–313). New York: Routledge, Taylor & Francis Group.

Hilgard, E.R. (1974). Toward a neo-dissociation theory: Multiple cognitive controls in human functioning. *Perspectives in Biology and Medicine*, 17, 301–316.

Hilgard, E.R. (1977). Divided consciousness: Multiple controls in human thought and action. New York: John Wiley & Sons.

Lyubomirsky, S., & Tkach, C. (2004). The consequences of dysphoric rumination. In C. Papageorgiou & A. Wells (Eds.), *Depressive rumination: Nature theory and treatment* (pp. 21–41). Chichester: John Wiley & Sons, Ltd.

Nolen-Hoeksema, S. (2004). The response styles theory. In C. Papageorgiou & A. Wells (Eds.), *Depressive rumination: Nature, theory and treatment* (pp. 107–123). Chichester: John Wiley & Sons, Ltd.

Papageorgiou, C., & Wells, A. (2001). Positive beliefs about depressive rumination: Development and preliminary validation of a self-report scale. *Behavior Therapy*, 32, 13–26.

Purdon, C. (2004). Psychological treatment of rumination. In C. Papageorgiou & A. Wells (Eds.), *Depressive rumination: Nature, theory and treatment* (pp. 217–239). Chichester: John Wiley & Sons, Ltd.

Rachman, S. (1997). A cognitive theory of obsessions. *Behavior Research and Therapy*, 35, 793–802.

Rachman, S. (1998). A cognitive theory of obsessions: Elaborations. *Behavior Research and Therapy*, 36, 385–401.

Sanders, D., & Wills, F. (2005). *Cognitive therapy: An introduction* (2nd ed.). London: Sage Publications.

Wegner, D.M., Schneider, D.J., Carter, S.R., & White, T.L. (1987). Paradoxical effects of thought suppression. *Journal of Personality and Social Psychology*, 53, 5–13.

Wells, A. (1990). Panic disorder in association with relaxation induced anxiety: An attentional training approach to treatment. *Behavior Therapy*, 21, 273–280.

Wells, A. (2000). *Emotional disorders and metacognition: Innovative cognitive therapy*. Chichester: John Wiley & Sons.

Wells, A., & Papageorgiou, C. (2004). Nature, functions, and beliefs about depressive rumination. In C. Papageorgiou & A. Wells (Eds.), *Depressive rumination: Nature, theory and treatment* (pp. 3–20). Chichester: John Wiley & Sons, Ltd.

Wenzlaff, R.M. (2004). Mental control and depressive rumination. In C. Papageorgiou & A. Wells (Eds.), *Depressive rumination: Nature, theory and treatment* (pp. 59–77). Chichester: John Wiley & Sons, Ltd.

# Behavioral Activation Therapy

Depression often occurs as a reaction to adverse life events such as the break-up of a relationship, the death of a loved one, loss of a job, or serious medical illness (Hammen, 2005). A study by Frank, Anderson, Reynolds, and Ritenour (1994) revealed that 65% of people with depression reported a negative life event in the 6 months prior to the onset of their depression. Moreover, people with depression are more likely to than nondepressed people to have chronic life stressors, such as financial strain or a bad marriage, and these people also tend to have a history of traumatic life events, particularly events involving loss (Hammen, 2005). These observations led Lewinshon and Gotlib (1995) to propose the behavioral theory of depression, which suggests that life stress can lead to depression by reducing positive reinforcers in a person's life. As a result, the depressed person begins to withdraw, causing further reduction in positive reinforcers, leading to more withdrawal, and thus creating the self-perpetuating cycle of depression. Therefore, it is not surprising that depression is characterized by feelings of sadness, misery, and a sense of apathy, resulting in pervasive impairment of the capacity to experience pleasure or to respond positively to the anticipation of pleasure. Such inhibitions of the mechanism of pleasure lead to diminished interest and investment in the environment. Consequently, depressed patients are unable to enjoy or participate in once pleasurable activities such as hobbies, eating, sex, or social interaction. In this chapter, I describe behavioral, physical, and hypnotherapeutic methods for dealing with avoidance and inactive behaviors. The methods include (a) techniques for dealing with avoidant behaviors, (b) physical exercise, (c) active–interactive training, and (d) hypnotherapeutic strategies for dealing with avoidance behaviors.

## TECHNIQUES FOR DEALING WITH AVOIDANT BEHAVIOR

According to Lewinshon and his colleagues (1974, 1986), when behavior decreases due to nonreinforcement, other symptoms of depression such as low energy and low self-esteem are likely to follow. In general, research has provided some support for the behavioral theory of depression (e.g., Rehm & Tyndall, 1993). Similarly, Rehm (1977) described depression as a deficit state characterized by lack of adaptive self-reinforcement. However, Willner (1991) believes the neurobiological changes accompanying prolonged stress may underpin such dampened hedonic capacity, and therefore the fundamental problem may be decreased reward salience rather than decreased exposure to rewarding activities. This view complements Seligman's (1975) learned helplessness model of depression. To counteract behavioral inactivation and avoidance, the *weekly activity schedule* and *behavioral activation training* are used.

Behavioral techniques are combined with CBT to counteract the behavioral inactivation component of depression, which includes anhedonia, lethargy, and lack of motivation. Friedman, Thase, and Wright (2003) have proposed a useful guiding principle for using behavioral technique within the CBT framework. They suggest that the greater the degree of the patient's behavioral inactivation, the greater the need for using behavioral techniques. The behavioral activation strategies include activities scheduling, graded task assignments, and mastery-pleasure exercises. These techniques help to actively overcome the lethargy cycle of depression, in which amotivation and indecisiveness, fatigue, lethargy, and anhedonia reinforce the automatic negative thoughts and beliefs of inadequacy and failure. This cycle becomes self-reinforcing, because worry and inactivity lead to sleep-cycle disintegration, which promotes further biological dysregulation that compromises the subjective appraisals of well-being (Friedman, et al., 2003). Friedman et al. believe behavioral techniques ameliorate both the behavioral and the biological components of the depression.

## Weekly Activity Schedule

An effective way to reverse this cycle is to utilize the *weekly activity schedule* (see Appendix 13A), which engages the patient in planned activities that substantially increase access to reinforcement. The weekly activity schedule is a calendar-like template that allows the patient to document how he spends time and to schedule activities. The patient is instructed to fill in the hourly grid with his activities and, in the next session, the therapist reviews the activities the patient engaged in over the past week. The patient is taught to appraise realistically the mastery and pleasure experienced while performing these activities. In so doing, the patient comes to see that an adequate degree of mastery can be achieved even when little pleasure is derived from an activity. Conversely, some activities, in the absence of complete mastery, can also be very pleasurable. By self-monitoring his hedonic capacity with the weekly activity schedule, the patient learns how expectations and predictions lead to specific mood states and behavioral outcomes. Martell (2003) has listed several reasons for using the weekly activity schedule:

• It reveals the patient's level of activity.
• It highlights restrictions imposed by negative mood.
• It shows the connection between activity and mood.
• It provides ratings for mastery and pleasure.
• It assists the patient in monitoring avoidance behaviors.
• It facilitates guided activity.
• It underscores steps the patient is taking to achieve stated life goals.

## Behavioral Activation Training

Although the weekly activity schedule can help depressed patients increase daily activities, some patients still continue to avoid some activities or situations. Behavioral activation training

**APPENDIX 13A:    Weekly Activity Schedule**
**Date: Week Starting_____ Week Ending_____**
**Please grade activities M for mastery and P for pleasure and**
**rate them on a scale of 0–10; 0 = no mastery or pleasure and**
**10 = full mastery or pleasure; Monday 9–10 and 10–11**
**completed as examples**

| Time | Monday | Tuesday | Wednesday | Thursday | Friday | Saturday | Sunday |
|------|--------|---------|-----------|----------|--------|----------|--------|
| 8–9 | Got out of bed M7 | | | | | | |
| 9–10 | Read P8 | | | | | | |
| 10–11 | | | | | | | |
| 11–12 | | | | | | | |
| 12–13 | | | | | | | |
| 13–14 | | | | | | | |
| 14–15 | | | | | | | |
| 15–16 | | | | | | | |
| 16–17 | | | | | | | |
| 17–18 | | | | | | | |
| 18–19 | | | | | | | |
| 19–20 | | | | | | | |
| 20–21 | | | | | | | |
| 21–22 | | | | | | | |
| 22–23 | | | | | | | |
| 23–24 | | | | | | | |

(BAT) provides a strategy for helping patients change their behaviors in such a way as to bring them into contact with positive
reinforcers in their natural environment. However, for such treatment to succeed, the therapist must take an idiographic approach.
Merely applying broad classes of pleasant activities may not be
reinforcing to every depressed patient, and thus a good functional
analysis is required. BAT is adapted from Martell (2003), and it
consists of three steps for dealing with avoidance. These steps
are illustrated by three acronyms utilized by Martell: ACTION,
TRAP, and TRAC.

ACTION stands for *assess, choose, try, integrate, observe*, and
*never*.

- *Assess:* The patient examines the current behavior and assesses
  whether it is avoidant behavior or whether it will serve to
  achieve a goal.

- *Choose:* The patient chooses to engage in the current behavior or to avoid it. The patient determines whether engaging in this behavior will help overcome depression in the long run.
- *Try:* The chosen behavior is tried out.
- *Integrate:* The new activity is integrated into regular routine. However, the patient reminds himself that trying a new behavior once is unlikely to lead to significant change.
- *Observe:* The patient observes the outcome of the new behavior. Specifically, the patient observes the impact of behavioral activation on mood and improvement in a life situation.
- *Never:* The patient decides not to give up in the face of disappointments. The patient realizes that counteracting depression and avoidance behaviors requires continued work.

TRAP stands for *trigger, response*, and *avoidance pattern*.

- *Trigger* can be an event or a situation.
- *Response* is the patient's emotional response to the trigger.
- *Avoidance pattern* is the typical avoidance response to the trigger.

Once the patient has identified a TRAP, the third acronym is used to get back on TRAC. TRAC stands for *trigger, response*, and *alternative coping* (instead of avoidance, alternative coping strategies are used in response to the trigger).

The bulk of the techniques for dealing with avoidant behavior are devoted to coaching depressed patients on how to use the activity charts, recognize avoidance pattern, and modify avoidance behaviors. Activity scheduling and avoidance work are particularly helpful in the initial stages of CBT. When working with these techniques, the therapist should adopt a collaborative stance. The therapist serves as a coach and helps the patient understand the areas of his life that are not working and to make adjustments in behavior to enhance the chances of reaching life goals. To enhance mastery and accomplishment of these tasks, the patient is helped to formulate realistic goals, based on realistic expectations of abilities. Realistic expectations can be deduced from activities that were successfully completed in the past. However, they should be modified to match the current depressive state of the patient. Therefore, tasks and assignments should be designed to re-establish self-efficacy. This can be done in a graded manner, slowly increasing the complexity and difficulty of the tasks assigned to the patient in proportion to both his ability and the degree of improvement in the depression.

## PHYSICAL EXERCISE

When patients have made some improvement (usually after around eight to ten sessions), they are encouraged to start some sort of physical exercise. Physical exercise has the capacity to prevent mental illness, foster positive emotions, and buffer individuals against the stresses of life (Mutrie & Faulkner, 2004). There is a convincing body of evidence in support of the strong relationship between physical activity and psychological well-being (Biddle, Fox, & Boutcher, 2000). In fact, the strongest evidence for the role of physical activity in promoting psychological functioning comes from the area of depression. Four epidemiological studies have demonstrated that lack of physical activity increases the risk for developing clinical depression (Camacho, Roberts, Lazarus, Kaplan, & Cohen, 1991; Farmer, Locke, Moscicki, Dannenberg, Larson, & Radloff, 1988; Paffenbarger, Lee, & Leung, 1994; Strawbridge, Deleger, Roberts, & Kaplan, 2002). Although the role physical activity in the treatment of mental illness has long been recognized, it is only recently that that the idea has been subjected to empirical investigation. Again the most compelling evidence comes from studies in the area of clinical depression. Two meta-analyses reported effect sizes of 0.72 (Craft & Landers, 1998) and 1.1 (Lawlor & Hopker, 2001) for exercise, compared to no treatment for depression. These effects sizes were comparable to other psychotherapeutic interventions. Moreover, one study showed the effect of 16 weeks of exercise to equal the effect of a standard antidepressant drug (Blumenthal, et al., 1999). At 6-month follow-up, there was some indication that those who continued to exercise had additional benefits compared with those patients on medication (Babyak, et al., 2000). In fact, the National Health Service in the United Kingdom has listed on their web site exercise as one of the treatments that may be helpful to people with depression (May 03, http://cebmh.warne.ox.ac.uk/cebmh/elmh/depression/new.html). There is consistent evidence from meta-analyses, randomized control trials, and large-scale epidemiological surveys that physical activity can make people feel better (Biddle, et al., 2000). Feeling good during and/or after physical activity can serve as a motivational spurt for other activities.

Chapter 16 further discusses the benefits of physical exercises with depression. Paterson (2002) believes exercise alleviates depression by creating a sense of exhilaration or euphoria ("runner's high"), which produces improvement in mood, increases energy, and reduces stress. Paterson considers regular physical exercise to be the cheapest and most effective physical treatment for depression. He recommends either *aerobic* or *anaerobic* exercises for depression. An exercise is considered aerobic if it raises the heart rate into a specified target range for a specified period of time. Such activities as running, swimming, cross-country skiing, and aerobics are considered aerobic exercises. Activities such as yoga, tai chi, and walking are considered anaerobic or nonaerobic because these exercises are not designed to raise the heart rate or sustain the heart rate for a specified length of time.

When prescribing physical exercise, depressed patients often wonder if they have the time, energy, or resources to exercise regularly. These concerns can become a justification for avoidance. Paterson (2002) provides several strategies for dealing with such avoidance.

- Get a physical. The patient must check with his physician for any limitations regarding physical exercises before starting.
- Pick the right activities. The biggest challenge is not to give up. It is important to pick activities that are easy, enjoyable, and that can be practiced at a convenient location.
- Variety helps. Select more than one activity and alternate among them. Choose activities for both summer and winter.

Experiment with a new activity. If it's not suitable, switch to another.

- Stretch and warm up first. Learn to do stretching exercises properly, and always do them before starting each exercise session. It is also important to do some low-intensity warm-up activities first before going into the main exercises. For example, before jogging, start with a brisk walk and gently break into a jog.
- Frequency is more important than duration. Regular short periods of exercises are better than irregular long periods. Exercise three to four times a week for about 30 to 60 minutes each session.
- Focus on enjoyment. Depressed patients who exercise for enjoyment and challenge seem to show greater improvement in mood than those who exercise to look better. The emphasis should be on how you feel, not how you look.
- Nothing changes overnight. Set an achievable and realistic goal when planning your fitness program. For example, start with low-intensity jogging for 15 minutes, rather than committing yourself to job 3 miles daily.

Compliance can also be increased by educating the patient and sharing the scientific findings of the link between exercise and depression. On occasion, referring the patient to a personal trainer in the local gym or health club proves helpful.

### ACTIVE–INTERACTIVE TRAINING

When interacting with their internal or external environment, depressed patients tend to dissociate to their inner reality (areas of concerns) rather than actively interacting with the relevant external information. *Active–interactive training* is utilized to break this pattern of interaction with the environment (Alladin, 1994, 2006). Active interaction means being alert and "in tune" with the incoming information (conceptual reality), whereas passive dissociation is the tendency to anchor in "inner reality" (negative schemas and associated syncretic feelings), which inhibit reality testing or appraisal of conceptual reality. Active–interactive training instructs patients on how to break away from their dissociative habits and associate with the relevant environment. To prevent passive dissociation, a person must (a) become aware of such a process occurring, (b) actively attempt to inhibit it by switching attention away from "bad anchors," and (c) actively attend to relevant cues or conceptual reality. In other words, the patient learns to actively engage the left brain hemisphere by becoming analytical, logical, realistic, and syntactical.

Active–interactive training can be illustrated by describing how Martin learned to interact actively with his environment. Martin is a 40-year-old married man with a history of recurrent depressive disorder. He believes his depression results from emotional and physical abuse he was subjected to from his father. This occurred over several years during his childhood. Martin has lots of anger and resentment towards his father, and he tends to ruminate a great deal about his unhappy childhood. Martin complains about his inability to focus or concentrate on simple daily activities: "I can't even watch TV, I can't read, or even have a conversation. I zone out, my mind is not here. I'm in my house, my father screaming at me." Martin was coached to recognize this as passive dissociation and to teach himself to be mindful of the present and aware of what he is doing (while watching TV, he reminds himself of the name of the program, the story line, and why he likes this program). After a week of training, Martin was able to break his dissociative habit and interact more actively with his conceptual reality, thereby increasing his ability to problem solve.

## HYPNOTHERAPY FOR ENHANCING BEHAVIORAL ACTIVATION STRATEGIES

Chapter 4 discussed the *response styles theory of depression* (Nolen-Hoeksema, 1991, 2004), which conceptualizes rumination as repetitive and passive thinking about symptoms, possible causes, and consequences of the depression. Depressed patients have the tendency to become preoccupied with catastrophic thoughts and images in response to a stressor. Several studies (see Papageorgiou & Wells, 2004) have provided evidence that depressed patients, compared with nondepressed individuals, ruminate for longer duration, exert little effort to problem solve, express lower confidence in problem solving, and have greater orientation to the past. According to the response styles theory, depressive rumination exacerbates and prolongs symptoms of depression, and aggravates moderate symptoms of depression into major depressive episodes. This form of rumination is conceptualized as a form of negative self-hypnosis (NSH) within the circular feedback model of depression (CFMD). As discussed in Chapter 4, NSH can easily lead to dissociation.

Dissociation occurs when one part of a person's mental or physical experience functions distinctly or independently from another part (Edgette & Edgette, 1995, p. 145). Within the context of depressive rumination, dissociation refers to the sense of detachment from the immediate physical environment and the events taking place in it that the depressed person experiences. However, dissociation is not always counterproductive; it can also be productive or adaptive. In fact, the dissociative phenomenon can be utilized as a technique for dealing with unadaptive dissociation. Dolan (1991) and Edgette and Edgette (1995) describe a number of ways to help patients convert the symptom of dissociation into a resource for healing. Hypnotherapy can be organized around helping patients learn to control their dissociation. With depression, dissociation can be a useful resource for those who get stuck in a sense of helplessness, hopelessness, and pessimism that erodes the core of the depressed person's self-esteem. Edgette and Edgette (1995) consider dissociation to act as a wedge between the depressed person's self-esteem (self-schema) and his present feeling about himself.

Edgette and Edgette (1995, pp. 145–158) describe several techniques for developing adaptive dissociation. For example, a patient with habitual maladaptive dissociation can be trained to adopt adaptive dissociation (Alladin, 2006), which helps to:

- Counter maladaptive dissociation
- Break the continuous pattern of negative rumination
- Halt the sense of pessimism and sense of helplessness

- Associate with success
- Integrate different parts of the psyche
- Detach from toxic self-talk

Edgette and Edgette (1995, p. 149) provide an example of how to use dissociation to remove the "wedge" between negative self-schema and current emotional experience:

You can bring to mind the idea of this wedge. It can come to you in the form of image or of simply a concept, abstract to your conscious mind and exquisitely material to your unconscious. So that your unconscious can take this wedge, and begin to find the suitable placement, inside, softly, carefully resting the edge between that one part of you that has felt lost and hopeless, between this and that other part of you that has remained untainted by the sadness, left whole and hopeful still. And it can be this whole part that stays ... operative ... no matter what ... ascending ... separate and whole ... allowing you to function, and to heal.

The dissociative phenomenon can also be used to disengage the depressed patient from constant (almost obsessional) rumination on a sense of failure, sense of loss, and sense of worthlessness. While in trance, the patient is coached to become more associated with successes and less dissociated with personal failings and shortcomings, thereby creating a healthier mental balance. Similarly, forward projection can be used to associate more with future success than dissociating with past failures or losses (see Torem, 2006).

Hypnotherapy can also be utilized to increase compliance with the behavioral activation strategies described in this chapter. Forward projection, behavioral rehearsal, ego-strengthening, and posthypnotic suggestions are particularly helpful.

## SUMMARY

This chapter described several techniques for helping depressed patients deal with inactivity and avoidance behaviors. Behavioral activation training promotes exposure to positive reinforcements from the environment. Physical exercise has been found to be beneficial with depression, and patients are encouraged to exercise regularly. Depressed patients tend to dissociate to their inner reality. To counteract passive dissociation, patients are coached to interact actively with their environment. These activation methods are reinforced by hypnotherapy, thereby creating compliance.

## REFERENCES

Alladin, A. (1994). Cognitive hypnotherapy with depression. *Journal of Cognitive Psychotherapy: An International Quarterly*, 8(4), 275–288.

Alladin, A. (2006). Cognitive hypnotherapy for treating depression. In R. Chapman (Ed.), *The clinical use of hypnosis with cognitive behavior therapy: A practitioner's casebook* (pp. 139–187). New York: Springer Publishing Company.

Babyak, M., Blumenthal, J.A., Herman, S., Khatri, P., Doraiswamy, M., Moore, K., et al. (2000). Exercise treatment for major depression: Maintenance of therapeutic benefit at 10 months. *Psychosomatic Medicine*, 62, 633–638.

Biddle, S.J.H., Fox, K.R., & Boutcher, S.H. (2000). *Physical activity and psychological well-being*. London: Routledge.

Blumenthal, J.A., Babyak, M.A., Moore, K.A., Craighead, E., Herman, S., Khatri, P., et al. (1999). Effects of exercise training on older patients with major depression. *Archives of Internal Medicine*, 159, 2349–2356.

Camacho, T.C., Roberts, R.E., Lazarus, N.B., Kaplan, G.A., & Cohen, R.D. (1991). Physical activity and depression: Evidence from the Alameda County Study. American *Journal of Epidemiology*, 134, 220–230.

Craft, L.L., & Landers, D.M. (1998). The effect of exercise on clinical depression resulting from mental illness: A meta-analysis. *Journal of Sport and Exercise Psychology*, 20, 339–357.

Dolan, Y.M. (1991). *Resolving sexual abuse: Solution-focused therapy and hypnosis for adult survivors*. New York: W.W. Norton.

Edgette, J.H., & Edgette, J.S. (1995). The handbook of hypnotic phenomena in psychotherapy. New York: Brunner-Mazel.

Farmer, M., Locke, B., Moscicki, E., Dannenberg, A., Larson, D., & Radloff, L. (1988). Physical activity and depressive symptoms: The NHANES 1 Epidemiological follow-up study. *American Journal of Epidemiology*, 128, 1340–1351.

Frank, E., Anderson, B., Reynolds, C.F., & Ritenour, A. (1994). Life events and the research diagnostic criteria endogenous subtype: A confirmation of the distinction using the Bedford College methods. *Archives of General Psychiatry*, 51, 519–524.

Friedman, E.S., & Thase, M.E. (2006). Cognitive-behavioral therapy for depression and dysthymia. In D.J. Stein, D.J. Kupfer, & A.F. Schatzberg (Eds.), *Textbook of mood disorders* (pp. 353–371). Washington, DC: American Psychiatric Publishing.

Hammen, C. (2005). Stress and depression. *Annual Review of Clinical Psychology*, 1, 293–320.

Lawlor, D.A., & Hopker, S.W. (2001). The effectiveness of exercise as an intervention in the management of depression: Systematic review and meta-regression analysis of randomized controlled trials. *British Medical Journal*, 322, 1–8.

Lewinshon, P.M. (1974). A behavioral approach to depression. In R.J. Friedman & M.M. Katz (Eds.), *The Psychology of depression: Contemporary theory and research*. Washington, DC: Winston-Wiley.

Lewinshon, P.M., Munoz, R.F., Youngren, M.A., & Zeiss, A.M. (1986). *Control your depression*. Engelwood Cliffs, NJ: Prentice Hall.

Martell, C.R. (2003). Behavioral activation treatment for depression. In W. O'Donohue, J.E. Fisher, & S.C. Hayes (Eds.), *Cognitive behavior therapy: Applying empirically supported techniques in your practice* (pp. 28–32). New York: John Wiley & Sons, Inc.

Mutrie, N., & Faulkner, G. (2004). Physical activity: Positive psychology in motion. In P.A. Linley & S. Joseph (Eds.), *Positive psychology in practice* (pp. 147–164). New York: John Wiley & Sons.

Nolen-Hoeksema, S. (1991). Responses to depression and their effects on the duration of depressive episodes. *Journal of Abnormal Psychology*, 100, 569–582.

Nolen-Hoeksema, S. (2004). The response styles theory. In C. Papageorgiou & A. Wells (Eds.), *Depressive rumination: Nature, theory and treatment* (pp. 107–123). Chichester: John Wiley & Sons, Ltd.

Paffenbarger, R.S., Lee, I.M., & Leung, R. (1994). Physical activity and personal characteristics associated with depression and suicide in American college men. *Acta Psychiatrica Scandinavica*, 89, 16–22.

Papageorgiou, C., & Wells, A. (2004). Nature, functions, and beliefs about depressive rumination. In C. Papageorgiou & A. Wells (Eds.), *Depressive rumination: Nature theory and treatment* (pp. 3–20). Chichester: John Wiley & Sons, Ltd.

Paterson, R.J. (2002). *Your depression map*. Oakland, CA: New Harbinger Publications, Inc.

Rehm, L.P. (1977). A self–control model of depression. *Behavior Therapy*, 8, 787–804.

Rehm, L.P., & Tyndall, C.I. (1993). Mood disorders: Unipolar and bipolar. In P.B. Sutker & H.E. Adams (Eds.), *Handbook of psychopathology* (pp. 235–262). New York: Plenum.

Seligman, M.E.P. (1975). *Helplessness: On depression, development, and death*. San Francisco: W.H. Freeman.

Strawbridge, W.J., Deleger, S., Roberts, R.E., & Kaplan, G.A. (2002). Physical activity reduces the risk of subsequent depression for older adults. *American Journal of Epidemiology*, 156, 328–334.

Torem, M.S. (2006). Treating depression: A remedy from the future. In M.D. Yapko (Ed.), *Hypnosis and treating depression: Applications in clinical practice* (pp. 97–119). New York: Routledge.

Willner, P. (1991). Animal models as simulations of depression. *Trends in Pharmacological Science*, 12, 131–136.

# Improving Social Skills

As noted several times before, major depressive disorder is characterized by impaired functioning in multiple domains, including biology, behavior, emotion, and cognition. Any of these domains can significantly affect the level of social functioning. The last chapter highlighted the behavioral theory of depression, which proposed that depression can result from the reduction of positive reinforcers and an increase in negative reinforcers in a person's life. One of the negative reinforcers is lack of social skills among depressed patients. *Social skills* are defined as the emission of behaviors which are positively reinforced by others. They involve the ability to communicate with other people in a fashion that is both appropriate and effective. Segrin (2000, p. 384) defines *appropriate behavior* as "social behavior that does not violate social and relational norms." Socially skilled behaviors are instrumentally effective because they allow successful achievement of goals in social situations.

Lewinshon (e.g., Lewinshon, 1974; Youngren & Lewinshon, 1980) has postulated that depressed patients, because of their lack of social skills, make it difficult to obtain positive reinforcement from the social environment and hence they become depressed. In Lewinshon's model, social skills deficits were viewed as an important antecedent to depression. Early studies of the theory provided consistent evidence that depressed patients exhibited poor social skills (Youngren & Lewinshon, 1980). However, longitudinal studies failed to support the hypothesis that poor social skills are direct causal antecedents to depression (Segrin, 2000). During the mid-1980s, this theory was integrated with cognitive theory, and the hypothesized relationship between social skills and depression was modified. Poor social skills were viewed as a consequence rather than a cause of depression. Only a few studies have examined the hypothesis that depression leads to lowered social skills, and the findings have been mixed. Therefore, a considerable degree of equivocality exists in the literature on social skills and depression. Segrin (2000), from his review of the relationship between social skills and depression, arrived at two conclusions. First, although poor social skills are concomitant to depression, no direct relationship between depression and social skills has been established because the relationship between depression and social skills is multiform. Second, poor social skills are not specific to depression; it is well-documented that people with schizophrenia, alcoholism, and anxiety also exhibit problems with social skills.

Whether poor social skills are antecedents or consequences of depression, the majority of depressed patients have interpersonal difficulties such as making friends, marital distress, low-frequency dating, a lack of close friends, insufficient social support, trouble initiating new relationships, strained relationship with coworkers, and impoverished social networks (Segrin, 2000). Moreover, social skills deficits may interact with other factors such as negative life events and operate as a risk factor for depression (Segrin, 2000). Furthermore, there is evidence that a particular instance of impaired social skills, known as *negative feedback seeking*, may also serve as a risk factor for depression (Joiner, 2002). Negative feedback seeking is defined as the tendency to actively solicit criticism and other negative interpersonal feedback from others. These propensities or diatheses reinforce the negative self-schemas of depressed patients. To modify this diathesis and to improve social skills, whether they are antecedents or consequences of depression, two to three sessions (or more if required) of cognitive hypnotherapy (CH) are devoted to teaching social skills training (SST).

## SOCIAL SKILLS TRAINING

In recognition of the pervasive association between social skills deficits and depression, social skills training (SST) is considered a very important component of CH. However, the decision to employ social skills training as an adjunct treatment is determined by the case formulation described in Chapter 6. The focus of this chapter is to describe a SST procedure adapted from Segrin (2003) that can be easily integrated with CH. Finally, the chapter provides some tips how SST can be amplified by behavioral rehearsal under hypnosis and posthypnotic suggestions.

SST is a generic term that refers to a number of specific forms of training such as assertion skills, conversational interaction skills, dating skills, and job-interviewing skills (Segrin, 2000). Table 14.1 summarizes some of the common SST techniques that can be easily integrated with CH.

The approaches to training these skills include instruction, modelling, rehearsal, role playing, and homework assignments outside of therapy sessions. Studies examining the effects of these trainings show clear improvements in social skills and self-reported measures of depression at 3- and 6-month follow-ups (Hersen, Bellack, & Himmelhoch, 1980). SST has also been found to be as effective as CBT, pharmacotherapy, and other forms of psychotherapy in the management of clinical depression (Bellack, Hersen, & Himmelhoch, 1981, 1983). Moreover, these studies showed significantly higher scores on measures of interpersonal skills and lower dropout rates for the social training group. The six techniques of SST summarized in Table 14.1 are briefly described next. These techniques can be easily integrated with CH, and the effects of SST can be amplified by hypnotherapy.

### Assessment for SST

Since social interaction skills are extensive and complex, it is important to take an idiographic approach. It is wrong to assume that all patients in need of SST will require the same type of intervention. Moreover, as noted before, SST is a nonspecific procedure, consisting of an amalgamation of techniques. Therefore it

**Table 14.1. Techniques utilized in social skills training (adapted from Segrin, 2003, p. 386)**

| Step | Descriptions |
| --- | --- |
| Assessments | Social skills deficits determined from case formulation, self-reports, behavioral observations, and/or third party. |
| Direct instruction or coaching | Explain the basis for appropriate and effective social behaviors and provide specific instructions to the patient on how to enact such behaviors. |
| Modeling | Model appropriate social behaviors and encourage the patient to enact these behaviors; provide positive reinforcements for doing so. Modeling, enactment, and critiquing of inappropriate behaviors can also be helpful. |
| Role-playing | Patient is encouraged to practice certain social behaviors in a controlled environment, such as with the therapist or an assistant. Provide feedback to the patient immediately after the role-playing. |
| Homework assignments | Patient is instructed to enact certain social behaviors in the real world. Start with easy behaviors and gradually progress to more complex behaviors. Review and provide feedback in the next session. |
| Follow-up | Reassess the patient's progress and, if necessary, calibrate the social skills. |

is essential to conduct an assessment before starting the training. The assessment will indicate what type of social skills training is required. In the absence of a proper assessment, resources may be expended on teaching skills that the patient already possesses and missing skill areas in which the patient genuinely needs improvement.

Social skills can be assessed by a variety of methods. The case formulation approach described in Chapter 6 provides a structure within which social and interaction skills training can be easily assessed. Therapists are encouraged to use the Cognitive Hypnotherapy Case Formulation and Treatment Plan from Appendix 6A in their initial assessment of the patient. The subsections *Interpersonal difficulties*, *Occupational problems*, *Leisure activities*, *Precipitants and activating situations*, *Strengths and assets*, and *Obstacles* force the therapist to explore the social skills of the patient. Here's an example of the information derived from Mary, from an assessment of her interpersonal difficulties (see completed example of Cognitive Hypnotherapy Case Formulation and Treatment Plan in Appendix 6B):

Interpersonal difficulties:
*She is socially isolated, avoids friends and social events. She has good social skills and several close women friends. She has never dated seriously, but she wants to marry and have children. Her friends from her office have, on several occasions, arranged for her to meet men, but she always declined their offers at the last minute. She believes she will never marry because she feels uncomfortable meeting men.*

From this assessment, it is apparent that Mary has good social skills, but lacks dating skills. The subsection *Early adverse negative life events* informs the therapist of the origin of Mary's unassertive behaviors: *"she became passive, fragile, and unassertive like her mother"* (see Appendix 6B). From this it would appear Mary is influenced by modeling behaviors. This serves as important information when the therapist selects SST techniques.

Another method of assessing social skills is to use self-report instruments. These instruments fall into two classes: those that assess social skills as a trait-like entity (e.g., Social Skills Inventory; Riggio, 1986, 1989) and those that measure particular components or aspects of social skills, such as the Conflict Resolution Inventory (McFall & Lillesand, 1971) or the Dating and Assertion Questionnaire (Levenson & Gottman, 1978). These instruments are psychometrically sound and very easy to use.

Social skills can also be assessed from behavioral observation. While this ideally entails naturalistic observation, staged role-play with the therapist or an assistant can provide an alternative context for observation. Information about social skills can also be obtained from third parties such as spouses, friends, coworkers, and so on. In the clinical setting, I find the case formulation approach adequate for assessing social skills in my depressed patients. However, I will use self-rating, observational, and third-party assessment if the need arises.

### Direct Instruction and Coaching of Social Skills

Having decided on the target for intervention, the next step is to offer concrete instructions on how to interact more effectively with people. Within the CH framework, this is achieved by one-on-one conversation with the patient. The patient is provided instructions on how to use various communication behaviors effectively, substantiated by giving a rationale for how and why certain behaviors are effective and appropriate. The following excerpt from Segrin (2003, p. 387) provides an example of how the therapist can utilize direct instruction, coaching, and explanation for showing interest in other people:

The social skills trainer might start by stating that showing interest and paying attention to our conversational partners make them feel valued. Further, most people respond very positively to others who make them feel worthwhile, valued, and cared for. The latter information provides an explanation for how and why showing interest in others works, and how it can be functional. In direct instruction and coaching the trainer must explain how to enact the behaviors and how they work to create rewarding social interactions and relationships. The therapist might offer suggestions for how to show interest in other people. "How's it going today?" and then following up with another inquiry or a positive response to what the other person has to say. Similarly the therapist might suggest that the client ask questions such as "How was your weekend?" or "What have you been up to lately?" Of course, it would be important to work on developing these conversation starters in more extended interactions in which the client responds appropriately to the discourse of his or her partner. These suggestions would be coupled with discussions and explanations of their effect on other people (e.g., making them feel valued, letting them know that other people care about them, and so on).

## Modeling Social Skills

Human beings predominantly acquire new behaviors through modeling (Bandura, 1977). Hence, it is not surprising that therapists utilize modeling as an important component of SST. Liberman and colleagues (1989) argue that modeling and imitation are the most effective methods of teaching complex social behaviors. The purpose of modeling is to demonstrate the effective and ineffective use of certain behaviors. In CH, the therapist usually acts as the model. When depressed patients have difficulty saying or doing certain things in the presence of others, they feel more comfortable doing them after seeing someone else perform the behaviors first. Modeling works because it gives the depressed patient a template or guide for her own behavior (Segrin, 2003). Bandura (1986, p. 66) refers to this as "making the unobservable observable"; that is, people cannot observe their own behavior, but once they have observed others' behavior, it gives them a mental picture of how to behave. It thus gives them a perceived *response of efficacy*; the feeling that this task can be accomplished. Response efficacy is an important component in reducing anxiety in social situation; hence, it has the ability to increase approach behavior and enhance social reinforcement in depressed patients.

## Role-Playing Social Skills

Coaching and modeling are passive techniques for learning social skills. For social skills training to be integrated in the repertoire of a patient's behaviors, active and interactive training is important. Role-playing provides the context for practicing the actual behavior learned and modeled. The purpose of role-playing is to have the depressed patient practice the desired behaviors in a controlled and safe setting, in which she can be observed and provided feedback and reinforcement. On occasions, a patient must role-play several times until the desired responses are produced.

## Homework Assignments

Homework assignments provide the patient with the opportunity to practice targeted behaviors in real situations. When assigning homework, it is important for the therapist to prepare the patient for failures. The therapist explains that it is unrealistic to expect success in every social interaction and that the goal of SST is simply to increase the probability of success in social situations. It is also important to review the homework assignments during the next session and provide supportive feedback and reinforcement.

# 15

# Mindfulness and Acceptance

Depression involves withdrawing or turning away from experience to avoid emotional pain (Germer, 2005). Such withdrawal can deprive the depressed person of the life that can only be found in direct experience. Germer believes successful therapy outcome results from changes in a patient's relationship with his particular form of suffering. For example, if a depressed patient decides to be less upset by events, then his suffering is likely to decrease. But how do we help a depressed person become less upset by unpleasant experiences? The previous chapters described a variety of techniques for modulating negative experience. This chapter focuses on mindfulness and acceptance—radical, but simple techniques for becoming less reactive to negative events in the present moment.

## MINDFULNESS IN PSYCHOTHERAPY

In recent years therapists from various clinical orientations have been utilizing mindfulness-based procedures to help depressed patients challenge their depressive stance. Mindfulness is a very simple way of relating to experience. It is based on the teaching of Buddha and Buddhist psychology. Buddha attributed human suffering to the tendency to cling to thoughts, feelings, and ingrained perceptions of reality and habitual ways of acting in the world (Lynn, Das, Hallquist, & Williams, 2006). In contrast, mindfulness directs one's attention to the task at hand. When mindful, one's attention is not entangled in the past or the future, and one is not judging or rejecting what is occurring at the moment. One *becomes* the present; this kind of attention can generate energy, clear-headedness, and joy (Germer, 2005). Most people with psychological disorders are preoccupied with past or future events. Particularly, the depressed person has a tendency to become preoccupied with feelings of guilt, regret, and sadness related to past events, or to constantly ruminate on future suffering. In such a scenario, the person strays from the present moment and becomes absorbed in past or future suffering, resulting in the exacerbation of depression. The person thus becomes the depression. As described in Chapter 4, this process is not dissimilar to negative self-hypnosis (NSH). Germer (2005, p. 5) provides a very lucid description of this:

As our attention gets absorbed in mental activity and we begin to daydream, unaware that we are indeed daydreaming, our daily lives can become a nightmare. Some of our patients feel as if they are stuck in a movie theatre, watching the same upsetting movie their whole lives, unable to leave. Mindfulness can help us to step out of our conditioning and see things freshly—to see the rose as it is.

Mindfulness helps us to be less reactive to what is happening now. As a result, our overall level of suffering is reduced and our sense of well-being increases. However, it is important to note that when a mindfulness approach is utilized in therapy, the therapist is not invalidating the patient's past history and is not unrecognizant of the fact that depression is a biopsychosocial-spiritual disorder. The narrative history of a person struggling with depression can be critically important: What happened in the past can bear on the present pain. For these reasons, mindfulness and acceptance are introduced during therapy or after acute-phase treatment. It is important to have already worked with triggering or maintenance factors and to have addressed issues related to the past or the future before taking a mindfulness approach in therapy. It is also important to have established a strong positive alliance so that the patient does not feel that her past history and the complexity of her depression is undermined.

Although mindfulness occurs naturally, its maintenance requires practice. There are two types of mindfulness training: formal and informal. *Formal* mindfulness training involves mindful mediation, allowing practitioners the opportunity to experience mindfulness at its deepest levels. *Informal* mindfulness training refers to the application of mindfulness skills in day-to-day living. Any exercise such as paying attention to one's breathing or listening to ambient sounds in the environment can alert us to the present moment; with acceptance, this cultivates mindfulness. In the therapeutic context, informal mindfulness is usually taught with the goal of helping patients disengage from their disruptive patterns of thinking, feeling, and behavior, and experience the relief of moment-to-moment awareness. For example, Teasdale, Segal, and Williams (1995) developed a mindfulness-based cognitive therapy (MBCT), utilizing acceptance and meditation, to help patients distance themselves from depressive ruminations. MBCT combines aspects of CBT with some components of the mindfulness-based stress reduction (MBSR) program developed by Kabat-Zinn (1990) and his colleagues. Unlike MBCT, which is a generic program applicable to a variety of problems, MBCT is specifically designed by Teasdale and his colleagues to treat unipolar depressed patients who are in remission. Unlike CBT, in MBCT little emphasis is placed on changing the content of thoughts; rather, the emphasis is on changing awareness of and relationship to thoughts, feelings, and physical sensations (Segal, Teasdale, & Williams, 2004). MBCT is an 8-week relapse prevention group treatment for depressed patients who are successfully treated with CBT or medication, or a combination of both. Patients are trained to defocus away from the content of their thinking and to direct their attention to the thinking process. They are coached in becoming aware of the occurrence of their thoughts without responding to them emotionally and without examining the accuracy of their beliefs. This approach teaches depressed patients to learn to separate themselves from feelings and thoughts and not to consider them as objective facts. An emotion or a thought is regarded as simply a behavior, a part of the person, and not the whole person. This ability to distance or *decenter* away from a cognition or affect aids patients in maintaining control over their thoughts (prevents catastrophizing) and feelings (mutates negative affect).

MBCT was empirically evaluated in a three-center study (Teasdale, Segal, Williams, Ridgeway, Soulsby, & Lau, 2000) involving 145 patients, with at least two previous episodes of major depression (77% had experienced three or more episodes), in remission or recovery, randomly assigned to treatment as usual (TAU) or MBCT. All the patients who participated in the study were previously treated with antidepressant medication but had been symptom-free and off medication for at least 3 months before entering the trial. Compared to the TAU group, MBCT reduced relapse rate by 44% in the group of depressed patients with three or more episodes of depression at 60 weeks follow-up, after the end of the 8-week program. In contrast, the relapse rate in the TAU group increased over the study period in a statistically significant linear relationship with number of previous episodes of depression: two episodes, 31% relapse/recurrence; three episodes, 56% relapse/recurrence; and four or more episodes, 72% relapse/recurrence. Similar results were found in a replicated study of depression (Ma & Teasdale, 2004). The investigators attribute the success of MBCT with depressed patients to decreased overgeneralized memories and ruminative thinking.

## MINDFULNESS-BASED HYPNOTHERAPY

Mindfulness can be easily integrated with hypnotherapy in the management of depression. Lynn, Das, Hallquist, and Williams (2006, p. 145) suggest that "hypnosis and mindfulness-based approaches can be used in tandem to create adaptive response sets and ameliorate maladaptive response sets." They recommend using hypnosis to catalyze mindfulness-based approaches. Since meta-analytic studies, qualitative reviews, and controlled trials have shown hypnosis to enhance the effectiveness of both psychodynamic and cognitive behavioral psychotherapies (Kirsch, 1990; Kirsch, Montgomery, & Sapirstein, 1995; Bryant, Moulds, & Nixon, 2005; Alladin, 2005; Alladin & Alibhai, 2007), it is reasonable to expect that hypnosis will also enhance the effectiveness of mindfulness training.

### Mindfulness-based Training in Cognitive Hypnotherapy

Mindfulness training is introduced to the depressed patient near the end of CH sessions (around Session 15). I find the following sequential training of mindfulness helpful to the depressed patients: first, education; second, training; and third, hypnotherapy. These three components of mindfulness training are briefly described next.

### *Education*

The patient is given an account, citing experimental evidence, of the risk factors involved in the exacerbation, recurrence, and relapse of depression, particularly after the acute-phase treatment or when the illness is in remission. Then, different strategies for relapse prevention are discussed, emphasizing the simplicity and effectiveness of mindfulness training. Once the patient agrees to mindfulness training, the complexity of the human being is discussed and, within this context, it is emphasized that feelings and thoughts are *part* of a person, not the whole self. It is pointed out that feelings and thoughts are not objective reality: They are impermanent, they come and go—like a cloud, while the sky stays the same.

## Training

The training involves *informal* mindfulness training consisting of the Body Scan Meditation exercise adapted from Segal, Williams, and Teasdale (2002, pp. 112–113). The patient is provided with a script of the Body Scan Meditation.

### Body Scan Meditation

1. Lie down on your back on a mat on the floor or on your bed. Assume a comfortable posture and allow your eyes to close gently.
2. Take a few moments to get in touch with your breathing and the feelings in your body. Become aware of the movement in your belly, feeling it rise or expand gently with every inbreath, and fall or recede with every outbreath. On each outbreath, allow yourself to let go or sink on the mat or the bed.
3. Become aware of the physical sensations in your body, noticing the sensation of touch or pressure in your body where it makes contact with the mat or bed.
4. Remind yourself of the reasons for this practice. Your intention is not to feel any different, but to become aware of any sensation you detect as you focus your attention on each part of your body in turn. You may or you may not feel calm or relaxed.
5. Now bring your attention to your lower abdomen. Become aware of the physical sensations in your abdominal wall as you breathe in and breathe out. Stay connected with your abdominal wall for a few minutes, attending to the sensations and feelings as you breathe in and out.
6. Now move your focus or "spotlight" of your awareness from your abdomen down to your left leg, into your left foot and all the way down to the toes of your left foot. Become aware of the sensations in the toes, maybe noticing the sense of contact between the toes, a sense of tingling or warmth, or no particular sensation.
7. Now you can move the spotlight to the breathing itself. Every time you breathe in, imagine the breath entering your lungs, travelling down into your left leg and left foot, all the way into the toes of your left foot. Every time you breathe out, you notice the outbreath leaving your toes, moving up your left foot and leg, into the abdomen and through your chest, all the way up, out through your nose. Continue breathing down into and out of your toes. This may appear difficult, but do the best you can and approach it playfully.
8. The next step is to let go of the awareness in the toes and to focus on the bottom of your left foot, becoming aware of the sensations in the sole of your foot, the instep, and the

heel, perhaps noticing the sensation in your heel where it makes contact with the mat or bed.

9. With the breath in the background, now allow your awareness to expand into the rest of your foot—into the ankle, the top of your foot, and right into the bones and joints. As you take a slightly deep breath, allow your awareness to move to the lower part of your left leg—into your calf, shin, knee, and so on in turn.

10. Now continue to bring your awareness to the physical sensations in each part of the rest of your body in turn—to the right toes, right foot, right leg, pelvic area, back, abdomen, chest, fingers, hands, arms, shoulders, neck, head, and face. It's not important how well you do, just do your best. Just continue to bring the same detailed level of awareness to the bodily sensation present. As you leave each area, "breathe in" to it on the inbreath and let go of the region on the outbreath.

11. When you become aware of any tension or intense sensations in any part of your body, just "breathe in" to them. Use your inbreath gently to bring your awareness right into the sensations and have a sense of release or let go on your outbreath.

12. From time to time your mind will wander away from your breath and your body. This is normal. This is what the mind does. So when you notice your mind wandering, just notice it, gently acknowledge it, notice where it has gone off to, and gently return your awareness to the part of the body you intended to focus on.

13. After scanning your whole body in this way, spend a few minutes being aware of a sense of your body as a whole and your breath flowing in and out of your body.

14. While practicing, if you find yourself falling asleep, you may prop up your head by using a pillow, or you may practice sitting up.

To increase compliance with the exercise, it is important that the patient is aware of the core aims of mindfulness training. Prior to starting the training, as part of the education, I go over the four core aims articulated by Segal, Williams, and Teasdale (2002, p. 86):

- To help depressed people learn skills to prevent their illness from recurring
- To develop awareness of different bodily sensations, feelings, and thoughts occurring from moment to moment
- To help develop a different way of relating to thoughts, feelings, and sensations. More specifically, to learn to accept and acknowledge unwanted feelings and thoughts rather than getting emotionally involved with them
- To develop the ability to choose the most skilful response to any unpleasant thoughts, feelings, or situation encountered

### Hypnotherapy

Lynn, et al. (2006) argue that basic instructions to practice mindfulness can be offered as hypnotic suggestions just as other imaginative or attention-altering suggestions. These scripts from Lynn, et al. (2006, p. 155) illustrate how hypnotic suggestions and images can facilitate mindfulness training:

Imagine that your thoughts are written on signs carried by parading soldiers (Hayes, 1987), or thoughts "continually dissolve like a parade of characters marching across a stage (Rinpoche, 1981, p. 53). Observe the parade of thoughts without becoming absorbed in any of them.

The mind is the sky, and thoughts, feelings, and sensations are clouds that pass by, just watch them (Linehan, 1993).

Imagine that each thought is a ripple on water or light on leaves. They naturally dissolve (Rinpoche, 1981, p. 44).

Lynn, et al. (2006) also recommend using hypnotic and posthypnotic suggestions to encourage patients to:

- Practice mindfulness on a regular basis
- Not to be discouraged when attention wanders off when training
- Learn to accept what cannot be changed
- Not to personally identify with feelings as they arise
- Learn to tolerate troublesome feelings
- Appreciate that troublesome feelings and thoughts are not permanent

The Body Scan Medication can be very easily integrated in the hypnotherapy session. An excellent hypnotic script for promoting acceptance and mindfulness can also be found in Lynn, et al. (2006, p. 155–156).

## ACCEPTANCE IN PSYCHOTHERAPY

Acceptance means receiving experience without judgment or preference, with curiosity and kindness (Germer, 2005a). Acceptance is not merely tolerance, it is the active nonjudgmental embracing of experience in the here and now, and it involves undefended exposure to thoughts, feelings, and bodily sensations as they occur (Hayes, 2004). Acceptance is utilized in psychotherapy to reduce distress by helping the distressed person notice different aspects of a situation or the relationship between the situation and the discomfort, or by creating a new stimulus that is less distracting or not distressing at all. This can be illustrated by describing how my friend, Ted, transformed his accident into creativity. Three years ago Ted, a child psychologist, was involved in a road accident in which he sustained a complicated fracture in his left foot. One evening, while he was riding his bike, he was hit by a motor vehicle. He fell off his bike and broke his foot. The driver was drunk. Ted had surgery, and he was off work for 4 months. Initially Ted was very angry with the driver, and felt it was very unfair that he should be hit by an irresponsible person, who did not care enough to refrain from drinking and driving. Ted ruminated on this scenario for about 3 weeks. Then he realized that there was nothing he could do about the accident and that it was a luxury for him to have several weeks away from work. He decided to utilize the time to write a paper on "affect regulation"—one that he had intended to write for a long time. Ted got so involved in his writing that he wrote two excellent papers that were accepted for publication. Ted's acceptance of the initial stimulus (accident) that was causing his distress was transformed into a different stimulus (writing) with different responses (preoccupation with writing, urgency to complete the papers, etc.). Ted still had thoughts about the drunken driver and the pain he was experiencing, but the pain and the accident were no longer the focal point for his energy and attention. Ted provides an example of pure acceptance. His goal per se was not to change his discomfort, but to utilize his time off the best way he could. In the process, the completion of his papers became the goal or target. Shifting Ted's attention to his writing might not have altered his experience of discomfort and displeasure, but he felt more content and productive.

Acceptance is also intended to increase decentering. Some evidence suggests that acceptance-based interventions reduce experiential avoidance and facilitate behavior change. For example, Levitt, Brown, Orsillo, and Barlow (2004) examined the effects of acceptance versus suppression of emotions and thoughts in the context of a carbon dioxide challenge in a sample of 60 patients diagnosed with panic disorder. The results suggested that acceptance may be a useful intervention for reducing subjective anxiety and avoidance in patients with panic disorder.

### Sense of Gratitude in Cognitive Hypnotherapy

I use sense of gratitude as a means of cultivating acceptance in my depressed patients. Although Western psychology has made remarkable progress in understanding the biopsychosocial roots of a troubled mind, it has neglected positive experiences such as well-being, contentment, love, courage, spirituality, wisdom, altruism, civility, and tolerance (Seligman & Csikszentmihalyi, 2000). We do not have a method for cultivating Olympic (advanced) levels of positive mental health (Germer, 2005). Moreover, the Western concept of the person and self emphasize separateness or individuality. In contrast, the non-Western concept of the person is embedded in the clan, society, and nature. Neither cultural concept is inherently better or worse than the other, just as no culture is good or bad. However, extreme cultural beliefs and values can create psychological problems. For example, Western society is very individualistic and preoccupied with ambition, success, and materialism. Although there is nothing wrong with having goals, ambitions, and consumer goods, it becomes a problem when people begin to attach their sense of worth, happiness, and fulfillment to these features and objects. Furthermore, Western society tends to emphasize that anyone can achieve anything he wants. This is unrealistic; a person cannot have everything he wants. Such belief and expectation often become the root cause of our "neurosis." Within this context, if a person does not achieve a goal, the person may see himself as a failure or worthless, often ending up with depression and a sense of hopelessness. These extreme values, by virtue of their lack of realism, are bound to produce failure. I (Alladin, 2006, p. 303) have given the example of a depressed patient who was not promoted at work and consequently started to ruminate on the beliefs that he is useless, worthless, and a failure. He believed that he "can never be happy," and "can't afford to buy whatever" he wants. Therefore:

"What's the point of going to work?" The patient was taught to be grateful for what he has, and hypnotherapy was utilized to reinforce this idea (see Alladin, 2006, p. 304).

This approach helps depressed patients prepare for dealing with loss, and it shifts their attention away from their minds to their hearts. If people can feel peace, harmony, and gratitude in their hearts, then they feel comfortable and satisfied mentally because people validate reality by the way they feel, not by the way they think. As with mindfulness training, cultivating a sense of gratitude also has three components: education, training, and hypnotherapy.

### Education

The patient is provided with a culture-neutral explanation highlighting some of the general differences between Western and non-Western societies in terms of culture, beliefs, values, and models of mind. The idea behind this exercise is to help the patient understand that values are subjective and culturally determined. It is expected that such understanding will help the patient to re-examine his meaning of life and appreciate that success and failure are culturally determined. The following cultural generalizations are emphasized:

- Different cultural values and beliefs
  - No culture is good or bad.
  - Cultural beliefs and values are learned and they differ from society to society.
  - Extreme cultural beliefs and values can create dysfunctional experiences and behaviors.
  - Therapists often act as agents to help depressed patients adopt a balanced view of "reality."
- Western expectation of life
  - Individuality or separateness is emphasized.
  - Individual success and material possessions provide respect.
  - Often means of achievement (legitimate or illegitimate) does not matter—success and material gain matter.
  - Success is tied to self-esteem and sense of worth.
  - When unsuccessful, low self-esteem, sense of failure, depression, hopelessness, and suicidal behavior are manifested.
  - Individuals are often brainwashed by unrealistic expectations such as "You can achieve anything you want," which sets up for failure.
  - When preoccupied with past or the future, we are not living in the present and not enjoying current resources.
- Non-Western expectation of life
  - Group, clan, or family identity is emphasized.
  - Respect for self is conditional on respect for family, group, and society.
  - Respect is based on meeting filial obligation.
  - Success depends on pleasing others.
  - When unsuccessful, the individual has group or family support.
  - Support and group identification reduce "neuroticism."
  - Extreme views, such as "take everything easy," may be dysfunctional.

- Western model of mind
  - Brain is the seat of existence.
  - Intellect and feeling are separate.
  - Most people don't know how to integrate intellect and feeling.
  - We validate reality by the way we feel.
- Non-Western model of mind
  - Heart is the seat of existence.
  - Feelings at heart validate reality.
  - Peace at heart provides peace of mind.

### Training

Depressed patients are encouraged to read books about different cultures and to begin to appreciate what they have. They are also instructed to write down five things they are grateful for everyday.

### Hypnotherapy

A sense of gratitude is easily integrated with hypnotherapy. This excerpt adapted from my work (2006, p. 303) illustrates how hypnotic suggestions can be crafted to reinforce sense of gratitude.

Just notice feeling calm, peaceful, and a sense of well-being. Feeling calm...peaceful...sense of harmony. No tension...no pressure...completely relaxed both mentally and physically...sense of peace...sense of harmony...sense of gratitude.

Become aware of your heart. Notice how peaceful you feel in your heart...you feel calm in your heart...you feel a sense of gratitude in your heart. When you feel good in your heart, you feel good in your mind.

All the major religions state that when you wake up in the morning, if you have a roof over your head, you have bread to eat, and water to drink, and is in fairly good health, then you have everything. Just become aware of all the things you have...all the things you are grateful for. It's okay to have goals and ambitions. When we achieve goals and ambitions, they are bonuses and pluses. When we don't achieve our goals and ambitions, it is disappointing, but we have enough resources to live a comfortable life.

### SUMMARY

Depression can recur or be exacerbated by negative experience or by ruminative depressive processing. The mindfulness and acceptance training described in this chapter provide two powerful techniques for regulating the depressive affect.

### REFERENCES

Alladin, A. (2005). *Cognitive hypnotherapy for depression: An empirical investigation*. Paper presented at the American Psychological Association Annual Convention, August 2005.

Alladin, A. (2006). Experiential cognitive hypnotherapy: Strategies for relapse prevention in depression. In M. Yapko (Ed.), *Hypnosis and treating depression: Advances in clinical practice* (pp. 281–313). New York: Routledge, Taylor & Francis Group.

Alladin, A., & Alibhai, A. (2007). Cognitive hypnotherapy therapy for depression: An empirical investigation. *International Journal of Clinical and Experimental Hypnosis*, in press.

Bryant, R., Moulds, M., Gutherie, R., & Nixon, R. (2005). The additive benefit of hypnosis and cognitive-behavioral therapy in treating acute stress disorder. *Journal of Consulting and Clinical Psychology*, 73, 334–340.

Germer, C.K. (2005). Mindfulness: What is it? What does it matter? In C.K. Germer, R.D. Siegel, & P.R. Fulton (Eds.), *Mindfulness and psychotherapy* (pp. 3–27). New York: Guilford Press.

Germer, C.K. (2005a). Teaching mindfulness in therapy. In C.K. Germer, R.D. Siegel, & P.R. Fulton (Eds.), *Mindfulness and psychotherapy* (pp.113–129). New York: Guilford Press.

Hayes, S.C. (2004). Acceptance and commitment therapy and the new behavior therapies: Mindfulness, acceptance, and relationship. In S.C. Hayes, V.M. Follette, & M.M. Linehan (Eds.), *Mindfulness and acceptance: Expanding the cognitive-behavioral tradition* (pp. 1–29). New York: Guilford Press.

Kabat-Zinn, J. (1990). *Full catastrophe living: Using the wisdom of your body and mind to face stress, pain, and illness*. New York: Dell.

Kirsch, I. (1990). *Changing expectations: A key to effective psychotherapy*. Pacific Grove, CA: Brooks/Cole.

Kirsch, I., Montgomery, G., & Sapirstein, G. (1995). Hypnosis as an adjunct to cognitive-behavioral psychotherapy: A meta-analysis. *Journal of Consulting and Clinical Psychology*, 63, 214–220.

Levitt, J.T., Brown, T.A., Orsillo, S.M., & Barlow, D.H. (2004). The effects of acceptance versus suppression of emotion on subjective and psychophysiological response to carbon dioxide challenge in patients with panic disorder. *Behavior Therapy*, 35, 747–766.

Lynn, S.J., Das, L.S., Hallquist, M.N., & Williams, J.C. (2006). Mindfulness, acceptance, and hypnosis: Cognitive and clinical perspectives. *International Journal of Clinical and Experimental Hypnosis*, 54, 143–166.

Ma, S., & Teasdale, J. (2004). Mindfulness-based cognitive therapy for depression: Replication and exploration of differential relapse prevention effects. *Journal of Consulting and Clinical Psychology*, 72, 31–40.

Segal, Z.V., Teasdale, J., & Williams, J.M.G. (2004). Mindfulness-based cognitive therapy: Theoretical rationale and empirical status. In S.C. Hayes, V.M. Follette, & M.M. Linehan (Eds.), *Mindfulness and acceptance: Expanding the cognitive-behavioral tradition* (pp. 45–65). New York: Guilford Press.

Segal, Z.V., Williams, J.M.G., & Teasdale, J.D. (2002). *Mindfulness-based cognitive therapy for depression: A new approach to preventing relapse*. New York: Guilford Press.

Seligman, M. & Csikszentmihalyi, M. (2000). Positive psychology: An introduction. *American Psychologist*, 55, 5–14.

Teasdale, J.D., Segal, Z.V., & Williams, J.M.G. (1995). How does cognitive therapy prevent depressive relapse and why should attentional control (mindfulness) training help? *Behavior Research and Therapy*, 33, 25–39.

Teasdale, J., Segal, Z.V., Williams, J.M.G., Ridgeway, V., Soulsby, J., & Lau, M.A. (2000). Prevention and relapse/recurrence in major depression by mindfulness-based cognitive therapy. *Journal of Consulting and Clinical Psychology*, 68, 615–623.

# Relapse Prevention

Although the majority of acutely depressed patients are success-fully treated either pharmacologically or psychologically, or with a combination of both, the current concern is that many of these successfully treated patients will relapse in the future. Follow-up research from across the globe is showing a return of new episodes of depression in people with a history of depression (Segal, Williams, & Teasdale, 2002) and the current alarming consensus is that relapse and recurrence is common among suc-cessfully treated depressed patients. For example, Paykel et al. (1995) found at least 50% of patients who recover from an initial episode of depression will have at least one subsequent depres-sive episode, and those patients with a history of two or more past episodes will have a 70% to 80% likelihood of recurrence in their lives (Consensus Developmental Panel, 1985). These find-ings led Judd (1997) to conclude that "unipolar depression is a chronic, lifelong illness, the risk for repeated episodes exceeds 80%, patients will experience an average of four lifetime major depressive episodes of 20 weeks' duration each" (p. 990).

These findings draw attention to the fact that relapse and re-currence following successful treatment of depression is common. Prior to these findings, relatively little attention was paid to de-pressed patients' ongoing risk. Now clinicians and therapists are beginning to make concerted effort to prevent recurrence and re-lapse in their depressed patients. Continuation treatment and on-going education regarding warning signs of relapse or recurrence are considered essential in ongoing clinical care. From the review of the literature, Dobson and Ottenbreit (2004) have identified three approaches for relapse prevention: (a) optimizing acute-phase treatment, (b) treating residual symptoms and mainte-nance treatment, and (c) developing specific relapse-prevention programs. Both pharmacological and psychotherapeutic strate-gies are used to optimize treatment during the acute phase in order to reduce the risk of relapse. Recently, hypnotherapy (see Alladin, 2006a) has been utilized to prevent relapses in depres-sion. Encouraged by the findings (Alladin, 2005, 2006; Alladin & Alibhai, 2007) that cognitive hypnotherapy (CH) produces larger effect size than cognitive behavioral therapy (CBT) in the man-agement of acute-phase depression and that patients from the CH group continue to improve after discharge, I (Alladin, 2006a) ex-panded the CH approach to actively deal with relapse prevention. I call this approach *experiential cognitive hypnotherapy* (ECH) be-cause it uses hypnosis and mindful techniques to help depressed patients decenter from negative feelings, images, and thoughts and search for nondepressive (mainly pleasant) affect. The rest of the chapter will describe how ECH strategies are used to

(a) optimize acute-phase treatment, (b) treat residual symptoms, and (c) provide maintenance treatment. The role pharmacological and other psychotherapeutic approaches is also highlighted.

## OPTIMIZING ACUTE-PHASE TREATMENT

The pharmacological approach focuses on either maintenance medication or having patients strategically cross over from one medication to another if the first medication does not work. Several follow-up studies (Belsher & Costello, 1988; Paykel, et al., 1999; Rafanelli, Park, & Fava, 1999) found that approximately 50% of depressed patients who are in remission or recovered from depression relapse following the discontinuation of either tricyclic antidepressants or selective serotonin reuptake inhibitors (SSRIs). On the basis of these findings the focus of drug treatment in depression has shifted from acute-phase treatment to long-term use of medication for maintenance. Prien and Kupfer (1986) found continuation treatment with antidepressants using the acute-treatment dose to be associated with reduced relapse rates compared to placebo. The optimal length of continuation treatment ranged from 4 to 9 months, and it was notable that a longer time of continuation therapy was not found to be more effective than placebo in preventing relapse (Reimherr, et al., 1998). Regarding the strategy of switching antidepressants, Koran, et al. (2001) found that more aggressive combinations of medication led to better clinical outcome and long-term prognosis than can be obtained from any single medication.

The main psychological approach utilized in the prevention of relapse in depression has been CBT. There is strong evidence that CBT has an enduring effect that reduces subsequent risk for relapse or recurrence following successful treatment (Hollon, Shelton, & Loosen, 1991). Several studies have shown that patients treated to remission with CBT are less likely to relapse after the termination of treatment than are patients treated to remission with medication (e.g., Blackburn, Eunson, & Bishop, 1986; Evans et al., 1992). Gloaguen, et al. (1998), from their meta-analysis of the effects of CBT for depression, concluded that CBT has better outcomes than medication: The average risk of relapse after CBT was 25% as opposed to 60% following pharmacotherapy at follow-up periods of 1 to 2 years. Dobson and Ottenbreit (2004) believe CBT produced better outcome because CBT effects lasting changes in negative cognitions, and it teaches depressed patients coping skills for dealing with stressors that may precipitate a relapse.

CH utilizes several strategies to optimize the acute-phase treatment to prevent relapse. These include:

- Systematic CBT
- Experiential hypnotherapy
- Cognitive restructuring under hypnosis
- Expansion of awareness and amplification of experiences
- Development of antidepressive pathways
- Reduction of guilt and self-blame
- Social skills training
- Physical exercise
- Preparation for discharge from acute-phase treatment

Most these strategies have already been described in Chapters 6 to 15. They are briefly described here to highlight how the strategies can be optimized during the acute-phase treatment to prevent relapse and recurrence of depression.

### Systematic Cognitive Behavioral Training

The effect of CBT can be optimized by making it as systematic as possible. At least four to six sessions of CH are devoted to CBT, or until the patient has mastered restructuring cognitive distortions using the ABCDE Form (see Chapter 8). It is important that the patient be able to identify, challenge, and correct dysfunctional beliefs that trigger depressive affect. Patients should be coached to differentiate between superficial ("I can't do this") and deeper (core beliefs) ("I'm a failure"), and they should be encouraged to constantly monitor and restructure their negative cognitions until it becomes a habit.

### Experiential Hypnotherapy

Hypnotherapy, particularly the hypnotic experience, provides a powerful placebo effect to the patient. The therapist can utilize and enhance this effect by inducing positive experience (by creating a pleasant state of mind) and by demonstrating the power of the mind through the cataleptic experience. Also as discussed in Chapter 8, ego-strengthening and posthypnotic suggestions should be realistic and specifically designed to counter rumination with negative self-hypnosis (NSH). As we (Alladin & Heap, 1991, p. 58) have indicated, ego-strengthening should be utilized to exploit "the positive experience of hypnosis and the therapist–patient relationship in order to develop feelings of confidence and optimism and an improved self-image." The reinforcement of positive affect and self-confidence bolster inner strength and prevent relapse.

### Cognitive Restructuring under Hypnosis

To consolidate the effect of cognitive restructuring under hypnosis, the experience must be "syncretic" (a matrix of affective, cognitive, somatic, and behavioral responses), and the cognitive restructuring must be repeated until a set of faulty cognitions related to a specific situation is considered to be successfully restructured (see Chapter 10).

### Expansion of Awareness and Amplification of Experiences

The effect of CH can also be optimized by expanding awareness and amplifying experience. This can be achieved by repeating the enhancing positive affective experience procedure (Brown & Fromm, 1990, pp. 322–324) (see Chapter 10) every time hypnosis is utilized in a treatment session. By intensifying positive feelings and creating awareness of various feelings, the procedure not only disrupts the depressive cycle but also helps to develop antidepressive pathways.

### Development of Antidepressive Pathways

Neuroimaging studies clearly indicate that CBT (Goldapple, et al., 2004) and hypnotic suggestions (Kosslyn, et al., 2000) can produce specific cortical changes in the brain. Within the CH context, positive imagery can be utilized to enhance the development of antidepressive or "happy" pathways (Schwartz, 1984). To optimize the development of antidepressive pathways, the therapist should attempt to amplify both the positive imagery and the associated somatosensory changes produced under hypnosis. Moreover, the technique should be repeated with at least three positive experiences and reinforced by posthypnotic suggestions (see Chapter 11).

## Reduction of Guilt and Self-blame

Depression can often be triggered or maintained by conscious or unconscious feelings of guilt and self-blame (old garbage). Chapter 10 describes several hypnotherapeutic techniques that can be used to reframe a patient's past experiences that cause present guilt or self-regret. The repetition of these techniques during acute-phase treatment with patients who express excessive guilt and self-blame can prevent preoccupation with guilt in the future.

## Social Skills Training

Social skills deficits may operate as a risk factor for depression under certain circumstances, such as in the presence of negative life events (Segrin, 2001). Moreover, evidence suggests that a particular instance of impaired social skills, known as *negative feedback seeking*, may also serve as a risk factor for depression (Joiner, 2002). Negative feedback seeking is defined as the tendency to actively solicit criticism and other negative interpersonal feedback from others. These propensities or diatheses reinforce the negative self-schemas of depressed patients. In order to modify this diathesis, two to three sessions (or more if required) of CH are devoted to teaching social skills, and the patient is advised to read the appropriate bibliography. The behavioral skills taught can be amplified by hypnotic behavioral rehearsal and posthypnotic suggestions.

## Physical Exercise

Chapter 13 reviewed the relationship between physical fitness and emotional health. Poor fitness is a risk for relapse in nondepressed individuals (Camacho, et al., 1991). On the other hand, physical exercise alleviates depression by creating a sense of exhilaration or euphoria ("runner's high"), producing improvement in mood, increasing energy, and reducing stress (Paterson, 2002). After six to eight sessions of CH, the patient is encouraged to get involved in some sort of physical exercise. To motivate the depressed patients to exercise, (a) the scientific findings of the link between exercise and depression are explained, (b) they are encouraged to join a gym or a health club, and (c) hypnotherapy is utilized to increase confidence via ego-strengthening, forward projection, and posthypnotic suggestions.

## Preparation for Discharge from Acute-Phase Treatment

Toward the end of the acute-phase CH (usually after 16 weekly sessions) when patients have been able to alter their deeper patterns of belief, affect, and behaviors, the last phase of the treatment is devoted to reinforcing the pattern of changes produced by the patients. The focus of the last few sessions of therapy is on setting realistic goals for the future. To increase confidence and create perceived self-efficacy of ideal but realistic future goals, hypnotherapy involving ego-strengthening, forward projection, and behavioral rehearsal is advisable.

## MANAGEMENT OF RESIDUAL SYMPTOMS

While the acute-phase treatment focuses on optimizing treatment to prevent relapse, the management of residual symptoms focuses on applying continuing treatment to patients who are in remission, but not fully recovered. Several pharmacological studies have provided evidence that the continuation of antidepressant medication reduce relapses in depression. For example, Glen, et al. (1984) demonstrated that 50% of their patients who were switched on to placebo after successful treatment relapsed compared to 20% of relapse in patients who continued with active medication. These findings led many clinicians to endorse the view that antidepressant medication should be prescribed prophylactically in order to prevent future episodes of depression. Unfortunately, the long-term use of medication presents several difficulties in terms of side-effects and other complications (see Alladin, 2006a). This led many clinicians to explore psychotherapeutic approaches for relapse prevention. A number of studies have provided support that the preventative effect of CBT is stronger than medication, with CBT relapse rates being consistently lower than those associated with continued medication (Dobson & Ottenbreit, 2004). For example, Fava, et al. (1994, 1996, 1998, 2004) reported on the long-term effect of CBT in patients who went into remission in response to antidepressant medication, but who continued to show residual symptoms. The relapse rates following CBT were 15% at 2 years, 35% at 4 years, and 50% at 6 years, while the relapse rates for the clinical management condition were 35% at 2 years, 70% at 4 years, and 75% at 6 years. Teasdale, et al. (2001) assert that CBT is more effective in relapse prevention than medication because CBT changes the manner in which previously depressed persons respond to negative thoughts. Based on these findings, I (Alladin, 2006a) developed several psychological strategies for treating residual symptoms of depression, including First Aid for Depression, Attention Switching and Positive Mood Induction, and Active–Interactive Training. After the completion of CH, patients with residual symptoms are encouraged to attend the clinic on a monthly basis for a year. During these sessions, some of the techniques used during the acute-phase treatment are reinforced and some new strategies are introduced.

### First Aid for Depression

The First Aid for Depression is fully described in Chapter 7. The technique can be reinforced whenever a patient experiences an exacerbation of her depressive symptoms elicited by environmental stressors. Moreover, patients are encouraged to practice, whenever upset, with the "cue word" to produce the good feeling associated with the First Aid technique (see Chapter 7).

## Attention Switching and Positive Mood Induction

Under conditions of stress, depressed patients tend to ruminate on catastrophic thoughts and images that may impede their therapeutic progress and lead to relapse. Chapter 11 described various techniques for breaking the negative ruminative cycle and creating more positive experiences. It is important to encourage patients to practice regularly using their positive experience list, at least once a day, because this is likely to turn negative self-hypnosis into positive self-hypnosis and strengthen the antidepressive pathways.

## Active–Interactive Training

Chapter 12 described the Active–Interactive Training technique for breaking dissociative habits and helping depressed patients associate with their relevant environment. Patients are encouraged to become aware of their maladaptive dissociation and to consciously adopt adaptive dissociation (Alladin, 2006a) to counter maladaptive dissociation and negative rumination. Such an exercise is likely to halt the sense of pessimism and helplessness and build associations with success.

## MAINTENANCE TREATMENT

The maintenance phase of treatment is developed to prevent fully recovered depressed patients from relapsing. After the termination of CH, these patients are encouraged to attend the clinic once a month for a year. Surprisingly, most patients are happy to continue with this phase of treatment because they see this as a preventative measure and an opportunity to consolidate the skills they have acquired during the acute-phase treatment. The focus of the maintenance phase is on:

- Enhancement of social connections
- Sense of gratitude
- Development of spiritual path
- Recognizing bias in thinking
- Catching and halting NSH
- Strengthening the antidepressive pathways

## Enhancement of Social Connection

Because human beings are social creatures, evolved to live in small communities, they do poorly when isolated. Hence, most human activities involve interaction with other people. Substantial evidence suggests that social support is a significant protective factor against the onset of depressive symptoms and that it aids in recovery (Lara, Leader, & Klein, 1997). In order to widen social contact and preserve social support, depressed patients are encouraged to broaden their social network. Paterson, et al. (1996) have provided three options for increasing the patient's social network. These include deepening current relationships, reviving old friendships, and starting new friendships. It is important for the therapist to provide their depressed patients full details and coaching on how to enhance each strategy for improving the social network. Hypnotherapeutic strategies such as future projection and behavioral rehearsal can be utilized to increase confidence and make the learning more experiential.

## Sense of Gratitude

Our Western society is very individualistic and preoccupied with ambition and materialism. Although there is nothing wrong with having goals, ambitions, and consumer goods, it becomes a problem when people begin to attach their sense of worth, happiness, and fulfillment to these features and objects. For example (Alladin, 2006a, p. 303), a depressed patient who indicates: "I can never be happy, I didn't get promoted. What's the point of going to work if I can't buy what I want?" is likely to be very unhappy at work and consequently may become depressed. Such a patient is taught to be grateful for what he has. Hypnotherapy can be utilized to reinforce this idea (see Alladin, 2006a, p. 304). This approach helps depressed patients prepare for dealing with loss, and it shifts attention away from the mind to the heart. If people can feel peace, harmony, and gratitude in their hearts, then they feel comfortable and satisfied mentally, because people validate reality by the way they feel, not by the way they think.

## Mindfulness and Acceptance

Recently, many clinicians have used mindfulness strategies to prevent relapse in depression. For example, Teasdale, Segal, and Williams (1995) developed a mindfulness-based cognitive therapy (MBCT) that draws on strategies from dialectic behavior therapy (acceptance and meditation) to help patients distance themselves from depressive ruminations. Patients are trained to defocus away from the content of their thinking and to direct their attention to the thinking process. They are coached to become aware of the occurrence of their thoughts without responding to them emotionally and without examining the accuracy of their beliefs. This approach teaches patients to learn to separate themselves from feelings and thoughts, and to regard an emotion or a thought to be simply a behavior, a part of the person, and not the whole person. This ability to distance or decenter away from a cognition or affect aids patients in maintaining control over their thoughts (to prevent catastrophizing) and feelings (to mutate negative affect).

## Development of Spiritual Path

Research suggests that people with religious faith or spiritual practice have lower rates of depression compared to those without religious or spiritual involvement (McCullough & Larson, 1999). Paterson (2002) found two aspects of spirituality to be helpful with depression: Privately held religious belief and practice, and involvement in a spiritual community, group, or organization focused on spiritual practice. The search for a spiritual community or the development of a spiritual path has been found to be particularly helpful to depressed people who have previously derived benefit from faith. Paterson (2002, p. 276) provides four suggestions for developing a spiritual path:

- Explore different faiths and practices until a particular faith or practice becomes meaningful.
- Sample different spiritual communities until one of them becomes appealing.
- If a religious-based community does not appear fulfilling,

consider other alternatives such as getting closer to nature by taking walks in the forest.
• Spirituality should not be seen as a prerequisite for overcoming depression; it should be pursued by people who feel comfortable with it.

### Recognizing Bias in Thinking

Patients are encouraged to become familiar with the 10 types of cognitive distortions (from Burns, 1999) listed in Chapter 2. The next step is to recognize distorted thinking and then to counteract this using "reminders" (see Alladin, 2006a, p. 306). For example, if a patient becomes aware of "disqualifying the positive," he reminds himself that "Positives too count—no excuses." Recognizing distorted thinking and counteracting it is akin to catching and halting negative rumination or NSH.

### Strengthening the Antidepressive Pathways

Patients are encouraged to practice regularly with positive mood induction exercises (see Chapter 11). Depressed patients who have been presenting vegetative symptoms (see Thase, et al., 1995, p. 7) during the acute phase of their depression are encouraged to use the positive mood exercise daily for a year.

### Self-Hypnosis

Many patients from the CH trial (see Chapter 3) reported that listening to their self-hypnosis audiotape daily was the most important factor in preventing the return of their depression. Therefore, in an attempt to prevent relapse, patients are encouraged to continue to listen to their self-hypnosis tape daily. They are also encouraged to utilize self-hypnosis techniques regularly until it becomes a habit.

### SUMMARY

The chapter described psychological strategies for preventing recurrence and relapse in depression. There is an urgent need to develop and evaluate various psychological programs, either alone or in combination with pharmacotherapy, to optimize the acute-phase treatment and to maximize residual and maintenance treatments. *Experiential cognitive hypnotherapy* (ECH) (Alladin, 2006a) offers a variety of treatment interventions for relapse prevention from which a therapist can choose the best-fit strategies for a particular phase of treatment. It also offers innovative techniques for becoming mindful of relapse and for developing antidepressive pathways. However, it is very important to evaluate the clinical effectiveness of ECH. It is only through appropriate evaluation that the effectiveness of ECH can be established.

### REFERENCES

Alladin, A. (2005). *Cognitive hypnotherapy for depression: An empirical investigation*. Paper presented at the American Psychological Association Annual Convention, August 2005.

Alladin, A. (2006). Cognitive hypnotherapy for treating depression. In R. Chapman (Ed.), *The clinical use of hypnosis with cognitive behavior therapy: A practitioner's casebook* (pp. 139–187). New York: Springer Publishing Company.

Alladin, A. (2006a). Experiential cognitive hypnotherapy: Strategies for relapse prevention in depression. In M. Yapko (Ed.), *Hypnosis and treating depression: Advances in clinical practice* (pp. 281–313). New York: Routledge, Taylor & Francis Group.

Alladin, A., & Alibhai, A. (2007). Cognitive hypnotherapy therapy for depression: An empirical investigation. *International Journal of Clinical and Experimental Hypnosis*, in press.

Alladin, A., & Heap, M. (1991). Hypnosis and depression. In M. Heap & W. Dryden (Eds.), *Hypnotherapy: A handbook* (pp. 49–67). Milton Keynes: Open University Press.

Belsher, G., & Costello, C.G. (1988). Relapse after recovery from unipolar depression: A critical review. *Psychological Bulletin*, 104, 84–96.

Blackburn, I.M., Eunson, K.M., & Bishop, S. (1986). A two-year naturalistic follow-up of depressed patients treated with cognitive therapy, pharmacotherapy and a combination of both. *Journal of Affective Disorders*, 10, 67–75.

Brown, D.P., & Fromm, E. (1990). Enhancing affective experience and its expression. In D.C. Hammond (Ed.), *Hypnotic suggestions and metaphors* (pp. 322–324). New York: W.W. Norton.

Burns, D. D. (1999). *Feeling good: The new mood therapy*. New York: Avon Books.

Camacho, T.C., Roberts, R.E., Lazarus, N.B., Kaplan, G.A., & Cohen, R.D. (1991). Physical activity and depression: Evidence from the Alameda County Study. *American Journal of Epidemiology*, 134, 220–230.

Consensus Development Panel (1985). NIMH/NIH consensus development conference statement: Mood disorders—Pharmacologic prevention of recurrence. *American Journal of Psychiatry*, 142: 469–476.

Dobson, K.S., & Ottenbreit, N.D. (2004). Tertiary intervention for depression and prevention of relapse. In D.J.A. Dozois & K.S. Dobson (Eds.), *The prevention of anxiety and depression: Theory, research, and practice* (pp. 233–260). Washington, DC: American Psychological Association.

Evans, M.D., Hollon, S.D., DeRubeis, R.J., Piasecki, J., Grove, W.M., Garvey, M.J., & Tuason, V.B. (1992). Differential relapse following cognitive therapy and pharmacotherapy for depression. *Archives of General Psychiatry*, 46, 971–982.

Fava, G.A., Grandi, S., Zielenzy, M., Rafanelli, C., & Canestrari, R. (1996). Four-year outcome for cognitive behavioral treatment of residual symptoms in major depression. *American Journal of Psychiatry*, 153, 945–947.

Fava, M., & Kaji, J. (1994). Continuation and maintenance treatments of major depressive disorders. *Psychiatric Annals*, 24, 281–290.

Fava, G.A., Rafanelli, C., Cazzaro, M., Conti, S., & Grandi, S. (1998). Well-being therapy. *Psychological Medicine*, 28, 475–480.

Fava, G.A., Ruini, C., Rafanelli, C., Finos, L., Conti, S., & Grandi, S. (2004). Six-year outcome of cognitive behavior therapy for prevention of recurrent depression. *American Journal of Psychiatry*, 161, 1872–1876.

Glen, A.I., Johnson, A.L., & Shepherd, M. (1984). Continuation therapy with lithium and amitriptyline in unipolar depressive illness: A randomized, double-blind, controlled trial. *Psychological Medicine*, 14, 37–50.

Gloaguen, V., Cottraux, J., Cucherat, M., & Blackburn, I.M. (1998). A meta-analysis of the effects of cognitive therapy in depression. *Journal of Affective Disorders*, 49, 59–72.

Goldapple, K., Segal, Z., Garson, C., Lau, M., Bieling, P, Kennedy, S., & Mayberg, H. (2004). Modulation of cortical-limbic pathways in major depression: Treatment-specific effects of cognitive behavior therapy. *Archives of General Psychiatry*, 61, 34–41.

Hollon. S.D., Shelton, R.C., & Loosen, P.T. (1991). Cognitive therapy versus pharmacology for depression. *Journal of Consulting and Clinical Psychology*, 59, 88–99.

Joiner, T.E., Jr. (2002). Depression in its interpersonal context. In I.H. Gotlib & C.L. Hammen (Eds.), *Handbook of depression* (pp. 295–313). New York: Guilford Press.

Judd, L.L. (1997). The clinical course of unipolar major depressive disorders. *Archives of General Psychiatry*, 54, 989–991.

Koran, L.M., Gelenberg, A.J., Kornstein, S.G., Howland, R.H., Friedman, R.A., DeBattista, C., et al. (2001). Sertraline versus imipramine to prevent relapse in chronic depression. *Journal of Affective Disorders*, 65, 27–36.

Kosslyn, S.M., Thompson, W.L., Costantini-Ferrando, M.F., Alpert, N.M., & Spiegel, D. (2000). Hypnotic visual illusion alters color processing in the brain. *American Journal of Psychiatry*, 157, 1279–1284.

Lara, M.E., Leader, J.B., & Klein, D.N. (1997). The association between social support and course of depression: Is it confounded with personality? *Journal of Abnormal Psychology*, 106, 478–482.

McCullough, M.E., & Larson, D.B. (1999). Religion and depression: A review of the literature. *Twin Research*, 2, 126–136.

Paterson, R.J. (2002). *Your depression map*. Oakland, CA: New Harbinger Publications, Inc.

Paterson, R.J., McLean, P.D., Alden, L.E., & Koch, W.J. (1996). *The Changeways core programme participant manual*, rev. ed. Vancouver Hospital and Health Sciences Centre, Department of Psychology.

Paykel, E.S., Ramana, R., Cooper, Z., Hayhurst, H., Kerr, J., & Barocka, A. (1995). Residual symptoms after partial remission: An important outcome in depression. *Psychological Medicine*, 25, 1171–1180.

Paykel, E.S., Scott, J., Teasdale, J.D., Johnson, A.L., Garland, A., Moore, R., et al. (1999). Prevention of relapse in residual depression by cognitive therapy: A controlled trial. *Archives of General Psychiatry*, 56, 829–835.

Prien, R.F., & Kupfer, D.J. (1986). Continuation drug therapy for major depressive episodes: How long should it be maintained? *American Journal of Psychiatry*, 143, 18–23.

Rafanelli, C., Park, S.K., & Fava, G.A. (1999). New psychotherapeutic approaches to residual symptoms and relapse prevention in unipolar depression. *Clinical Psychology and Psychotherapy*, 6, 194–201.

Reimherr, F.W., Amsterdam, J.D., Quitkin, F.M., Rosenbaum, J.F., Fava, M.F., Zajecka, J., Beasley, C.M., Michelson, D., Roback, P., & Sundell, K. (1998). Optimal length of continuation therapy in depression: A prospective assessment during long-term fluoxetine treatment. *American Journal of Psychiatry*, 155(9), 1247–1253.

Schwartz, G. (1984). Psychophysiology of imagery and healing: A systems perspective. In A. A. Sheik (Ed.), *Imagination and healing* (pp. 35–50). New York: Baywood.

Segal, Z.V., Williams, J.M.G., & Teasdale, J.D. (2002). *Mindfulness-based cognitive therapy for depression: A new approach to preventing relapse*. New York: Guilford.

Segrin, C. (2001). *Interpersonal processes in psychological problems*. New York: Guilford Press.

Teasdale. J.D., Scott, J., Moore, R.G., Hayhurst, H., Pope, M., & Paykel, E.S. (2001). How does cognitive therapy prevent relapse in residual depression? Evidence from a controlled trial. *Journal of Consulting and Clinical Psychology*, 69, 347–357.

Teasdale, J.D., Segal, Z.V., & Williams, J.M.G. (1995). How does cognitive therapy prevent depressive relapse and why should attentional control (mindfulness) training help? *Behavior Research and Therapy*, 33, 25–39.

Thase, M.E., Kupfer, D.J., & Buysse, D.J. (1995). Electroencephalographic sleep profiles in single-episode and recurrent unipolar forms of depression: 1. Comparison during acute depressive states. *Biological Psychiatry*, 1, 72–80.

# 17

# Future Directions

Hypnosis, in the realm of psychotherapy, has two major flaws: it does not provide a theory of personality or psychopathology, and its application (hypnotherapy) to the treatment of emotional disorders has not achieved the coveted status of well-established treatment. This chapter provides some future directions for increasing the credibility of hypnotherapy as an effective treatment for depression.

Since hypnosis does not provide a theory of personality and psychopathology, a theoretical framework for conceptualizing treatment is lacking and the manner in which hypnotherapy produces therapeutic outcome is very often not determined. As a rule, hypnotherapy has been used in a shotgun fashion or as an adjunct, without giving adequate attention to the disorder being treated and without stating how hypnotherapy per se will be used to alleviate the symptoms (Wadden & Anderton, 1982). In 1994, I (Alladin, 1994) made the first attempt to provide a conceptual framework, based on empirical, theoretical, and scientific rationale, for integrating hypnotherapy with cognitive behavior therapy (CBT) in the management of depression. This conceptualization has been revised and refined in this book (Chapter 4) as the *circular feedback model of depression* (CFMD). Although CFMD is not a comprehensive hypnotic theory of depression, it emphasizes the roles of negative self-hypnosis (NSH) and dissociation as important factors in the etiology of unipolar depression. However, CFMD should be further studied and refined, and this model can be used as an exemplar to develop other models of emotional disorders. For example, dissociation has been identified to be an important component in the development and persistence of posttraumatic stress disorder (PTSD) (see Lynn & Cardena, 2007). Further research should be conducted in this area, and a working model of PTSD comprising dissociation as a risk factor should be explored.

Hypnotherapy is not considered mainstream psychotherapy. Because several empirically supported treatments (e.g., CBT, interpersonal psychotherapy, and antidepressant medications) for clinical depression are available, why would a therapist utilize a treatment strategy, such as hypnotherapy, that has not been empirically validated? For hypnotherapy to be widely used and become accepted as a mainstream psychotherapy, its effectiveness must be demonstrated. Fortunately, several empirical studies, meta-analyses, and reviews clearly indicate that the treatment effect is enhanced when hypnotherapy is integrated with other forms of psychotherapy in the management of various emotional disorders. However, in none of these studies was hypnotherapy used as a stand-alone treatment; it served as an adjunct to a well-established psychotherapy, CBT in most cases. At present, in the area of emotional disorders, only two published randomized studies have demonstrated the superiority of cognitive hypnotherapy (CH) (hypnotherapy combined with CBT) over other forms of psychotherapy with emotional disorders.

The first study (Bryant, Moulds, Gutherie, & Nixon, 2005) compared hypnosis plus CBT with CBT and supportive counseling (SC) in acute stress disorder. Hypnosis plus CBT was better than the other two strategies for reducing the relapse of symptoms at the end of treatment. The second study (Alladin & Alibhai, 2007) reported in Chapter 5 compared CH with CBT. The results clearly indicated larger effect size for the CH group. These results confirm the findings and conclusions reported by Kirsch, Montgomery, and Sapirstein (1995) and Schoenberger (2000) that hypnosis in combination with CBT produces greater clinical improvements than CBT alone in the treatment of emotional disorders. Although these results are promising, the evaluation of the efficacy of CH is in its infancy. In the future, we need more comparative trials. Moreover, studies should be conducted to examine the effective components of hypnotherapy. For example, in the depression study (Chapter 5), CH consisted of *hypnotic induction, ego-strengthening, expansion of awareness, positive mood induction, posthypnotic suggestions*, and *self-hypnosis*. At this point, it is not clear which of these components increased the effect size.

Utilization of hypnotherapy in the management of depression has a bright future. However, for this promise to be fulfilled, research and evaluation are needed.

## REFERENCES

Alladin, A. (1994). Cognitive hypnotherapy with depression. *Journal of Cognitive Psychotherapy: An International Quarterly*, 8(4), 275–288.

Alladin, A., & Alibhai, A. (2007). Cognitive hypnotherapy therapy for depression: An empirical investigation. *International Journal of Clinical and Experimental Hypnosis*, in press.

Bryant, R., Moulds, M., Gutherie, R., & Nixon, R. (2005). The additive benefit of hypnosis and cognitive-behavioral therapy in treating acute stress disorder. *Journal of Consulting and Clinical Psychology*, 73, 334–340.

Kirsch, I., Montgomery, G., & Sapirstein, G. (1995). Hypnosis as an adjunct to cognitive-behavioral psychotherapy: A meta-analysis. *Journal of Consulting and Clinical Psychology*, 63, 214–220.

Lynn, S.J., & Cardena, E. (2007). Hypnosis and the treatment of posttraumatic conditions: An evidence-based approach. *International Journal of Clinical and Experimental Hypnosis*, 48, 154–169.

Schoenberger, N.E. (2000). Research on hypnosis as an adjunct to cognitive-behavioral psychotherapy. *International Journal of Clinical and Experimental Hypnosis*, 48, 154–169.

Wadden, T.A., & Anderton, C.H. (1982). The clinical use of hypnosis. *Psychological Bulletin*, 91, 215–243.

# Index

NOTE: Italic *f* indicates an illustration; *t* indicates a table.